SELF HELP AND MOVEMENT
FOR
RHEUMATIC SUFFERERS

SELF HELP AND MOVEMENT
FOR
RHEUMATIC SUFFERERS

WITH A
FOREWORD BY
COLONEL THE LORD LANGFORD O.B.E.

ALBERT BYRAM

ARTHUR H. STOCKWELL LTD.
Elms Court   Ilfracombe
Devon

ERRATA

Page 12, line 28
  for   butozoladine
  read   diphenylprazolidine
Page 131, line 3
  for   ... here is by finger and that
           precludes ...
  read   ... here is by finger and thumb, at
           the very end of the toe. There is
           one condition that precludes ...

ISBN 0 7223 1252-0
Printed in Great Britain by
Arthur H. Stockwell Ltd.
Elms Court   Ilfracombe
Devon

CONTENTS

Photographs set between pp. 64 & 65

FOREWORD
by
Colonel the Lord Langford, O.B.E.

I am one of Albert Byram's innumerable successes.

Many years ago now, I had a horrid fall when riding in a hurdle race and for some time afterwards I had intermittent and very painful back trouble. My then G.P., a personal friend who has since retired, advised me "to stop lifting heavy weights and to buy myself a heat lamp". He added that he would prescribe some pills.

When I asked if this was the best the great British Medical Profession could do for me, he replied that my back had suffered irreparable damage.

Not long afterwards and almost by chance, I had the profound good fortune to meet Albert Byram. Not only did he put right my back trouble within a month or two but, what is more, he and the advice he puts forward in this book have kept it right ever since, a period of over twenty years.

LANGFORD

Bodrhyddan
1 September 1977

PREFACE

This book is written mainly for the early rheumatic sufferer, but also for the person who desires to improve his general health and prevent the onset of rheumatism.

Prevention is always better than cure and RHEUMATISM is PREVENTABLE.

My most grateful thanks to all my patients who have not only supported me, but have taught me far more than all the text books. Also to all who have helped in the task of compiling this book:

To Miss Jean Davey who despite being severely handicapped typed the whole of my manuscript.

To Mr Arthur Parker who drew the difficult illustrations most wonderfully, without any previous artistic training, and after suffering two heart attacks.

To David Foden our superb wheelchair athlete for his modelling and smile, and to all the people in the future who give my methods fair trial.

Yours for health.

A. Byram

1

REASON FOR THIS BOOK

After fifty years of dealing with the rheumatic ailments, during which time I have given over a quarter of a million treatments, I feel that before I retire or pass on, it is almost a duty to endeavour to help some people to help themselves.

The views expressed in the following pages are founded on the results of many years of close observation, study, and hard work.

Some professional people may argue that there are slight discrepancies, I make no apologies — this book is not a medical text book — it is written mainly for the oft neglected sufferers.

Medicine has not been very successful in treating the rheumatic complaints, although surgery is doing wonderful work in the extreme and sometimes hopeless cases.

My main concern is with the people who have not yet reached the point of requiring surgery, and in the most neglected, but most important feature of rheumatism — PREVENTION. Allow me to examine a few of the things that have been done.

In general disease, great strides have been made by science and medicine, by better techniques, better hospitalization, new advances in medical apparatus, etc.

Many lives have been saved, and with improved hygiene, a better standard of living, plus the wonder drugs, penicillin, antibiotics, cytamen, etc.

Now we are living longer, but are we living better? We prolong life and often discover that the older person becomes stiffer and slower — in fact, rheumatism is well established in over 60% of people who have passed their 60th birthday.

Despite plenty of research the rheumatic diseases cost the country more and more each year; it now runs into hundreds of millions of pounds per annum, and what is more important, the suffering is getting steadily worse.

If by a different approach we could reduce this cost by only 15%, millions of pounds could be saved, and by using less drugs we could eliminate some of the dangerous side effects produced by these drugs. Let us now examine some of the efforts made by the medical profession.

The rheumatic research council conducted research many years ago, and concluded with the remark by Lord Holden (the then King's physician): 'We have *been unable to cure rheumatism*, because we have been unable *to find the cause*.'

More recently a famous professor, after many years of experiment and study, declared: 'We have tried everything for rheumatism — gold injections, silver injections, butozoladine, cortisone, A.T.C.H., etc., and not one has been better than the common aspirin, but they all have *dangerous* side effects.'

I well remember the huge headlines in the press 1949. CORTISONE IS PROVED A SURE CURE FOR RHEUMATOID ARTHRITIS. Like many of the other miracle cures it caused high hopes, that were dashed when the often terrible side effects came out. Far be it from me to belittle the medical profession, but in general doctors study disease, which is quite different from studying health.

This may sound somewhat strange to many people, but there are so many difficult studies in disease and about 30,000 different symptoms that the medico has little time to give to the study of health and nature. For nearly 60 years I have tried to learn how the body strives to keep healthy even under unhealthy conditions, and for most of that time my main interest has been in the rheumatic conditions. Many doctors have done their best to treat the rheumatic sufferers, but most patients want relief and demand drugs; what can the poor doctor do when he is overworked, overwhelmed, and probably suffering himself?

2

REASONS FOR ARTHRITIS

There have been many eminent people who have expressed concern about the enormous cost and suffering in the rheumatic field, but little effort has been made to reduce both in comparison with other diseases. The cost still rises yearly and more and more people become crippled. Over the years many things have been blamed for the onset of rheumatism, from getting cold, wet, hungry, to being attacked by a virus. In my humble opinion the main causes of rheumatism are OVERWORRY, OVERWORK AND OVER-EATING.

Many years ago the rheumatic patient was told to go to bed and rest, and even today this dangerous advice is still given. When there is a great deal of inflammation, or raised temperature, rest is certainly required, but as soon as this subsides, MOVEMENT IS VITAL.

Movement is life — stagnation is death.

Getting the upper hand and controlling your rheumatism is a fight, and the sufferer is advised by me to grit the teeth and move. There are drugs which relieve the pain, and many people take these, then as the pain subsides they sit back, (usually on a soft easy chair) and, doing nothing say "That's better", but it would be far better if when they felt easier they would get up and go.

This is the way to improvement — no doubt people have heard it said that going wears out the body — this is absolute rubbish — the body does not wear out — it *rusts out*, due to lack of movement. Muscles that are well used have a far better circulation, and even in middle age can grow stronger with exercise.

The recent photograph of your author, (book cover), in a finger stand, supporting the body weight on fingers that have been used extremely hard for over 50 years, surely proves that they have not worn out.

They can waste away with disease, they can become clogged with waste matter, they can rust, but never ever wear out. I am not particularly concerned with strength, but with freedom of movement, and whilst I agree that prime movers of joints are the muscles, every movement stimulates the bursa to lubricate the dry joint.

Bursa are wonderful glands situated around joints and tendons, not only to lubricate, but sometimes to act as a cushion between bones and tendons. There are twelve around the shoulder joint and they are all stimulated by warmth and movement.

Please consider this — is it not plain common sense that these glands tend to dry up, without movement, resulting in joints and tendons that have no lubrication? This could be the forerunner of arthritis. We can liken these dry joints to any rusty door hinge, creaking and groaning each time we open or close the door. What does one do with this rusty hinge? — oil it, then open and close the door many many times to rub off the rust and create a nice smooth hinge or joint.

Mr Charnley, the wonderful surgeon at Wrightington

Hospital, who was responsible for the early replace-
ment of arthritic hip joints by plastic ones said that
over 60% of these patients should never have required
this operation if only someone had given them
preventive advice. I now give it again — MOVE.
Even badly crippled people have some part of their
anatomy which is moveable — work on this — grit the
teeth, and in many cases one can so improve the
circulation that other parts start to loosen up.

I often wonder how much the present day style of
living has contributed to the increase in rheumatism.
There were so many occupations that were manual but
are now done by machine. What about the old-time
housewife, without electricity, vacuum cleaner, cooker,
and electric washer, who performed many exercises on
wash-day — scrubbing, possing, wringing, and even
filling the wash-tub with bucket after bucket of water.
Carpets were taken out into the garden or backyard,
and vigorously beaten with a bamboo beater or even a
hand brush. All the modern civilized gadgets have
taken most of the exercise out of life, and instead of
walking one tends to jump (or crawl) into the car.

The sedentary worker is in a sorry plight — off to
work in the car even if he works one mile away, back
home for evening meal, then off to the club or pub,
usually in the car again — almost total physical
stagnation. Add to this the present day traffic, the
mad rush of mental living and tension. No wonder
there is a great build up of acid in the body and
regretfully not enough physical work or exercise to use
up the damaging acid.

3

OVERWORRY AND ADRENALIN

Now to the main causes of rheumatism; the first without doubt is overworry. This builds acid into the system, and gradually destroys the chemical balance. When one worries, the suprarenal glands, aided by others, pump adrenalin into the bloodstream.

Adrenalin is acid, and it is a powerful stimulant, but also a poison. We can stimulate the flow of acid from our glandular system by our mental attitude, by getting angry, frustrated, depressed, and by worry. I would like to tell you of my first initiation of adrenalin.

In my early days my mother was a sufferer from rheumatoid arthritis, heart trouble and dropsy. We were very poor, and this, coupled with the struggles with Father, who returned from the 1914 war badly gassed and suffering from epileptic fits and nephritis, certainly affected Mother, who spent a large part of the next eight years in bed, and was relieved of her many troubles by gladly passing away at the age of 46.

In those days, particularly in the poor quarters, neighbours were always ready to help with cleaning, shopping or washing and we were blessed by a true helper, a fiery tempered little lady who hailed from London but settled unhappily in Oldham. Many times she roared into our little house, and as I watched in amazement, she cleaned the house with fantastic energy. At first I just couldn't understand where this slim, sickly-looking lady got her speed and strength from. One day she gave the clue by saying:

"I love to have a row then I can get through my work in half the time."

Today I really believe she caused a lot of trouble in our poor area just to feel the surge of adrenalin (not that she understood), but I was beginning to learn. My second lesson was a tragedy, and occurred at Moston colliery where two rippers aged around twenty were cutting a new tunnel through towards a fresh coal seam. Their job was to open the roof prior to the fitting of the pit props, and it certainly was both hard and dangerous. On this occasion part of the roof collapsed and a large part of the stone pinned one of the boys to the floor, breaking his pelvis, and he was slowly being crushed to death. His friend, in a terrible frenzy lifted the stone off and both boys were taken to hospital. Later the manager sent three men to remove the stone, but they found the task beyond them — obviously they couldn't secrete any adrenalin now that the excitement was over.

My family and I lived in one of a row of eight cottages which were sold in 1920, to a local tobacconist, for the sum of £100, not each, but for all the eight. My brother James had tuberculosis as an infant and was five before he could walk, however, with years of exercise, he won the 9 STONE BRITISH WEIGHT-LIFTING CHAMPIONSHIP at the age of forty.

For myself, at 14, I developed rheumatoid arthritis and was warned by our doctor not to move, "Otherwise you will be a cripple for life." Thank God I had just enough knowledge to ignore him. Some time later, Mother was sent to Buxton Hospital, then called the Royal Devonshire Hospital for rheumatism, and on my first visit I asked, "Who was the important man in the wheelchair?" Yes! You guessed it — he was the principal doctor. A further disturbing thought in those days was another poor man confined to a wheelchair, Mr J. Boots, the millionaire owner of Boots chemists. No doubt that these two gentlemen had had their worries, and perhaps generated plenty of acid, but we can surely learn from them.

Adrenalin is a very powerful substance which gives us temporary strength and terrific fighting power. The madman is using this when it takes six men to hold him down.

One of the greatest boxers of all time was an adrenalin fighter — in his early fights he would work himself into a real frenzy against his opponent, and before the start of the fight he would be fully charged with this secretion, which gave him greater speed, strength, and fighting power. This man was 'I am the greatest' MUHAMMAD ALI heavyweight champion of the world.

Because we have little control over our emotions we often lose our calm, and nature thinking we are suddenly in need of extra power, stimulates suprarenal glands to secrete adrenalin. This sudden call can damage the body if we don't understand what to do about this excess acid. Unless we quickly do some physical work or exercise, and use up this secretion, a residue is left in the bloodstream.

If you have had an argument with the chap next door and you feel het-up and rather trembly — it's adrenalin, and the best way to remedy this is to dig the garden or do any other physical task. The motto is that if you cause an adrenalin surge use it up by using your muscles. A better course is — don't encourage the secretion. Make an effort to combat worry, realize that worry cannot help, and it can certainly harm the body. Worry is negative and solves no problem.

I am aware that some people are almost born worriers, and it is difficult to stop, but if only you can learn one vital truth it must help. THIS IS IT — The body is always striving to maintain health, and given reasonable help we can all be healthier. I know perfectly well that drugs can save lives and often relieve pain, but drugs cannot make health. HEALTH IS TO BE WON BY A WAY OF LIVING, NOT BY A BOTTLE OF MEDICINE.

Years ago a famous doctor said, "Man recovers twice from disease, once from the disease and once from the medicine." Just recently, Doctor J.W. Riley of Telford, said: "If 80% of the drugs prescribed today were thrown into the sea only the fish would suffer."

Far be it from me to criticize your doctor. He has enough to do, with all the complications of illness, (many caused by present day living) and we have been taught to expect miracles from the profession, but the poor chap is only human. Try to take a little strain off him, by helping yourself to get a little nearer to nature. Eat more selectively, and less, move more, and above all endeavour to develop a calm and optimistic mind. The mind can break or make the body. There are times when it is necessary to see your doctor — any severe pain and unusual pain and prolonged inflammation, raised temperature, and in fact any doubtful condition, but remember, good health is your responsibility. I must stress again that the body does not wear out. IT RUSTS OUT, and many times the organs get so clogged with waste material that they can no longer function.

The joints of the body must have movement to prevent the rust from forming, and it is better to keep all the joints loose and free than to develop frozen shoulders, stiff knees, tight necks, and rigid spines. There are a few conditions of arthritic joints which have been started by trauma (injury) and afterwards neglected until there is no movement left — the only solution here is surgery, but to be undertaken only when all other methods have failed. Today we often hear the orthopaedic surgeon tell a patient that his broken limb, involving a joint, will certainly become arthritic in a few years. This is not necessary, if as soon as the plaster is removed treatment is begun with graduated massage and movement.

You ask — "Why don't they do this in hospital?" There are a few reasons why — they have insufficient time, often there are more urgent cases waiting, and the modern physiotherapist has gradually been weaned away from massage (maybe because it is hard work) and sometimes the patient is not prepared to attend for what may be long sessions, most of it waiting time.

4

LESSONS LEARNED FROM SUFFERERS

A wonderful insight into mental stress was a lady friend who suffered a most terrible skin disease, and had long periods in hospital under an eminent skin specialist, all to no avail. I had inspected this horrible skin, and suggested that besides her medical treatment she should go on a strict diet. Nothing doing, until one day she came to show me the incredible improvement in her skin — and all due to her spiritualism, she said! On enquiring how long she had been going to the spirits; she said, "Three months," but having some local knowledge I asked if it wasn't three months since her battleaxe of a mother-in-law, who lived with her, had died. "Oh yes Mr B., but I started to improve after the first meeting." REMOVE THE CAUSE AND THE EFFECT CEASES. The mind can make or break the body, and this is particularly true in rheumatism.

In my work I often find a regular patient who suddenly appears much worse, after steady gain, and now with increased pain and more difficult movement. Whilst massaging his muscles there is a much tighter tone, and a somewhat restricted circulation. After some conversation the cause often comes to the surface — the poor chap has had some bad luck financially, suffered a bereavement, or even as in one case, been burgled.

Again, we have the extra secretion of acid, plus extra pain, plus more difficult movement. This is what I call reverse circle, and our efforts must be to alter the direction from going backwards to going forwards. One cannot remain in one state of health or fitness; we either go backwards or forwards. Now if by treatment of various kinds we can reverse the backward circling to forwards, even a tiny little movement, we have gained, and once started in the right direction it will go forward with increasing momentum. So many sufferers allow their health circle to go backwards, due mainly to negative thinking, lack of movement, and the strange thought, 'I am getting old.' Because one is older in years it does not necessarily follow that one cannot improve. I have seen many people in their 70s and 80s improve enormously.

It has been my privilege to meet some wonderful people in my work and I certainly find that adversity builds character, which brings me to a wonderful lady, nearly 80 years young. I must report a little of Mrs Lewis, who battled on in a life mainly of pain which she endured with amazing courage and happy fortitude.

Despite many setbacks Mrs Lewis gritted her teeth, and pressed on against superhuman difficulties. What a privilege to know this super lady.

Mrs Lewis was married to a remarkable man, W.J. Lewis, B.Sc., who trained at Owen's College, now Manchester University, graduated in 1917 as an electro chemist, and joined a team which included Mr Rutherford, who first split the atom. Later W.J. Lewis went to Boots the chemist at Nottingham, making Lewis gas for war purposes. He had suffered from a congenital heart condition, and in the gas-making process, he developed arsenical poisoning, lost all his body hair, and became completely bald.

After the war he met his old college scientists, and having discovered a method of producing Amedol used in photography, he found sponsors in nobility with cash and faith. They established a laboratory on the site of an old colliery at Burslem, where electricity was on tap. They produced this chemical at a very competitive price and began business. Whilst alone on duty one night, Lewis slipped and fell into a vat of hydrochloric acid. Luckily there was a bath of water near by, and he managed to jump into this, but not before all his clothes and a lot of his skin burned off, leaving him naked and in great pain. Mr Lewis closed down the plant, donned the only garment he had (an old raincoat) and walked nearly a mile in the frost to his lodgings.

Shortly afterwards the German Government started to take an interest in this product, and, backed by State money produced Amedol at a much lower price. This was the time of the depression, and four scientists were out of work. Lewis tried to get a teaching position, but it was hopeless, and by this time he was suffering from chest trouble and pernicious anaemia, but he tramped the streets looking for work. Eventually he got a position with a builders' merchant in Oldham, married Mrs Lewis in 1924, then decided to branch out himself as a builders' merchant.

He rented a large yard from the council, and by living frugally made progress, helped by Mrs Lewis who did book-keeping and other work. Despite poor health he got the firm on a sound basis, and before he died aged 51 in 1948 of congenital heart disease the specialist said he thought that Lewis would have died in his teens.

During most of this period Mrs Lewis had been a sick woman weighing twelve stones, and suffering from arthritis, colitis, and thyroid trouble. Three weeks after her husband died, the local council gave Mrs Lewis notice to quit the business premises. Left with just two workers, Mrs Lewis decided to fight back at life's injustic and bought some rough land, set to work building sheds and a hut as an office, dealing in cement, plaster and heavy goods. She promised her two workers that if the business did well, she would promote them to directors, along with a niece, who had lived with her since being three years old.

Mrs Lewis worked really hard, even though she was always in pain, and the business prospered. At that time Mrs Lewis was the only female builders' merchant in Britain. In 1927 Mrs Lewis had her tail bone removed, in 1931 after working in the yard and unloading merchandise, she developed spastic colitis, and after three years' treatment, her weight was reduced to six stones and eight pounds. She suffered appendicitis in 1946, in 1947 a duodenal ulcer flared up, and the poor lady spent four weeks in a nursing home. After arriving home, she found her husband in bed with bronchitis. In 1957 a growth was removed from her throat and for five and a half years she had followed the specialist's advice, which was that she was not allowed to eat meat, vegetables, fruit or sweets. She existed mainly on two pints of milk daily with a tablespoonful of olive oil and Aludrox.

After Lewis died, Mrs Lewis worked hard until 1963, when she had a cardiac occlusion, and was in the intensive care unit under specialist Mr Janus for ten weeks. She went back to her book-keeping and accounting work, but in 1973 suffered another heart attack, and was tenderly treated by her own physician, Mr Livingstone. Later she became diabetic and her weight reduced from 12 stones to 8 stones 12 pounds.

She finished work at 75 years old, and began to do the things she enjoyed — painting, clay modelling, and getting out and about. She now says "Life is good" and she can enjoy a smooth relaxed rhythm with many hobbies and good friends. For many years I have treated this lady, and to say she amazes me is a great understatement. At 78 years of age she flew to Bahrain alone in the Concorde, a triumph of mind over matter and she had fantastic courage.

There is a great difference in people, and some give way (becoming non-triers). This can be disastrous, as the following example shows. I appreciate that fate is not kind to many people, and sometimes one can hardly blame them for giving way. Many years ago, a middle-aged lady came to see me. I knew her as a fairly close neighbour. With her hands and fingers curled up, and trembling a little, she informed me that she had arthritis in both hands. This is how the conversation ensued:

Albert: Have you seen your doctor?

Lady: No.

Albert: Who says you have arthritis?

Lady: I do, and the pain is terrible.

Albert: Have you ever had it before?

Lady: No.

Albert: Please take your gloves off.

Lady: I can't.

Albert: Who put them on?

Lady: I did.

Albert: Then take them off, it's far easier than putting them on.

After she removed the gloves I managed to get her into a more relaxed condition, and then I quietly moved every joint with ease whilst distracting her attention. Without doubt there was absolutely no sign whatever of any arthritis. The lady was obviously in a very nervous state, and on questioning her I discovered that she had had a very bad shock some four weeks previously, when her husband had gone completely blind. This was, as I know, enough to account for her nervous condition, but why only trouble in the hands? As I talked to her it slowly occurred to me that the worst feature of this tragedy was that the poor lady had acquired a terrible aversion to cutting her husband's food and meat, thus the fingers were objecting through her mind. Once again, the mind can make or break the body. I referred her to her doctor, and lost contact with her for about two years, by which time she was crippled with true arthritis all over her tragic body.

Another patient of mine whom fate helped to cripple via the mind was Alice. Alice had been a patient of mine for some years, nicely holding a reasonable degree of health and mobility, but after her husband Arthur became blind, and later when her son suffered a detached retina, Alice became arthritic in every joint.

Arthur came to me with osteo-arthritis in both hips; he was the least trouble of any patient I ever had. He had a quick wit, a sunny smile, and certainly knew his way about. In those days when we had bad fogs in this area, Arthur used to guide the sighted people home from the workshop for the blind after work. Once again we have the worry factor, as in so many homes, just like the arthritic lady with two mongol children; and Stanley's mother who struggled to give him the best she could for forty years without his father, who left him in infancy, totally spastic and quite unable to do anything for himself. Stan and I are great pals and I have been able to give him a little help during the past forty years. I could go on and on about so many of these afflicted people, but I want to record my personal view.

If I could wave a magic wand, and remove their worry overnight, 75% of these sufferers would be 75% improved by next morning. Of this statement I am 100% convinced. You may think I have stressed the worry angle too much, and what about the young children who develop rheumatism? I will just give one instance of a girl who had gold injections for arthritis at the tender age of five. When I treated her later it was soon apparent that the mind was again involved. This little girl had all the love of her parents until she was four years old, when a lovely baby boy was born, and I guessed that most of the love was transferred to him. This was the beginning of some resentment and frustration in the girl. Within eight months the poor girl was arthritic.

Shingles is considered by most medics to be caused by a virus related to chickenpox, but I had a regular rheumatic patient who came in one morning with a most dreadful shingle rash right down the sciatic nerve. Although her doctor called it a virus, she confided in me that three days previously she had her little granddaughter in the house, and unfortunately grandmother forgot to put the fireguard in front of the lounge fire. The little girl fell into the fire and was now in hospital. The poor grandmother naturally blamed herself and the resulting worry caused shingles and a sudden increase in her rheumatism.

5

OVERWORK

Whilst I have stressed the great importance of movement, I must warn against another cause of acid, namely overwork. When it is hard to continue working, and when one is very tired, by forcing the body to keep going is another way of creating acid. It is always a good thing to know when to ease off and rest, in fact, both in work and exercise one should always try to leave a reserve of energy if possible. Many ladies, after a hard day's work, will look around, perhaps late at night, see something that is not perfect, and say: "I am tired out, but I must get up and clean that carpet" (or whatever). This is overwork. One can work all day at an interesting job and not be tired, but forcing oneself to work when it becomes an unpleasant task creates acid as the body tires. In all effort always leave a reserve of strength, and train yourself to use the minimum of strength and energy in your work. If we are trying to build the body by exercise, we do the movements the hard way, using a great deal of effort; but in work, as we become more skilled, we conserve our energy and do our jobs with the minimum of strength and the maximum of skill.

Watch a craftsman in any trade, and we think 'That looks easy, I guess I could do that,' if we just try, we quickly find that it isn't easy. It is the skill of the operator which makes it appear easy.

So often the unskilled worker will lift, for example, a weight of two kilogrammes, and use enough strength to life twenty. This is due to fear of letting the object fall, or nervous tension, but with practise we can all use less power and do the task more smoothly and more easily, with less strain on our body and nerves. In watching an inexperienced man using a saw in his right hand, gripping far too tightly, we notice that his knuckles are white and tense, but just look at his left hand. This is just as tense as the right hand and many times his whole body is putting effort into the task and he is burning himself out. His left arm should be completely relaxed and hanging down into gravity with his fingers loosely open.

Whatever you are doing, think! 'Can I do this task an easier way? Am I relaxed enough? Am I doing a good job and gaining satisfaction from it? Is my breathing slow and easy? Am I standing or sitting with a good posture?' And most important, 'Can I take my mind off the pain and concentrate only on the work?' Pain is always worse when doing nothing. Find yourself a nice congenial task and a pleasant hobby to combat pain.

6

OVEREATING

Eating should be a pleasure, but please eat to live, not live to eat, and always leave the table while you are still hungry. Without doubt the greatest pleasure in life is *Good Health!* and I assure you it is not possible to have good health if you are overeating. Take some of the strain from the stomach by chewing your food well. Try not to drink with your meals. Drinking half an hour before meals is best.

Do not drink iced water with meals, particularly in hot climates. The stomach temperature should be the same as the body temperature, 98.4°, but if you take a cold drink with food this reduces the temperature of the stomach and digestion is delayed. In hot climates this delay can cause the food in the stomach to putrefy — which is particularly so at lunch-time when the outside temperature is high.

Whilst one is young and still growing more food is required and young, vigorous people can get along with some excess, but after 25 years of age we don't require half the amount of food, and for the sedentary worker even less is required. We can divide the body into roughly two types which require different amounts of food, and indeed thrive on different exercise. The two types of physical body with variations between them are:

TYPE A — (Fig. 1). Usually a fairly well-built body, often overweight, but the sign denoting the abdominal type is the high, wide rib cage. They prosper on fairly big meals with long intervals in between; two meals each day are usually best. They excel at slow endurance work, exercise and sport, and generally relax easily.

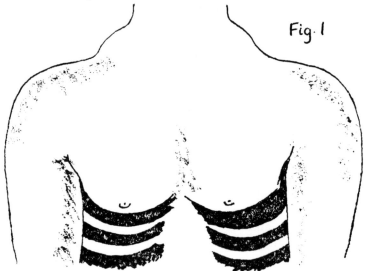

Fig. 1

ABDOMINAL TYPE

TYPE T — (Fig. 2). The thoracic type which has a narrow rib cage reaching to the hips. This type is usually better with six light meals each day. The stomach is usually much smaller than that of a Type A body. Food passes through their system much more quickly, and they gain less nourishment from it. They

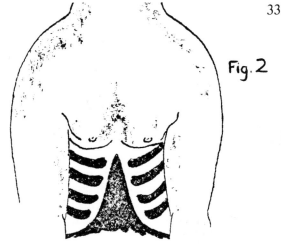

Fig. 2

THORACIC TYPE

don't put on weight, have great difficulty in relaxing, and tend to live on their nerves, but thrive on quick movements and should avoid endurance. As with food, so with exercise little and often, and rest in between is best

These are the greyhound breed. The body requires food and drink, but people do not realize how little is required to nourish the body, and what a wonderful and complicated process is digestion and assimilation. The hardest work man does is in the digestion of food; and to digest a big meal uses a fantastic amount of energy, far greater than, say, swinging a heavy sledge-hammer for hours. Shortly after eating a heavy meal more blood is called to the organs of digestion to help this vital process. This of course means that there is less blood in other parts of the body, particularly in the feet and brain, and certainly one shouldn't try to run just after a meal, neither can the brain function at

c

its maximum.

In grandfather's day, after his large Sunday lunch he got into his favourite rocking chair, and he was soon asleep, because all his energy was being used to digest his food and externally he was dormant. We can surely realize that if we take the strain off the digestion, we can also have more external energy. If we give it a trial by eating half as much and chewing our food more, eating more slowly, and not drinking with meals, not only will our food digest more easily and more quickly, but we will not have the usual bloated discomfort. Our food will be assimilated better, and give more nourishment than the bigger, less digested meal.

Give the stomach a chance. It is the most important organ in the body. Look after the stomach and the other organs will look after themselves. Quite a number of low back pains are caused by a distended lower bowel, and can be improved by better diet and exercise. If there is constipation, take more roughage in food, particularly All Bran, and eat more fruit, especially figs prunes and dates. Also drink one glass of water half an hour before meals.

If the trouble is flatulence, and this is very prevalent, check with your doctor that there is no ulcer, etc., and then reduce the stomach acidity, by not drinking with meals, but immediately afterwards, take half a glass of ice-cold milk slowly. Milk is a light protein and uses up some of the excess acid, which flows from the stomach. The cold drink contracts the glands and stops or slows down the acid flow. A hot drink opens the glands and stimulates a further flow of acid into an already over-acid stomach.

Whilst on the subject of food, there is one condition that aggravates arthritis and many other complaints.

This is the self-inflicted injury of *overweight*.

My advice is GET IT OFF! If you are overweight you are eating, or drinking, or both, more than your body requires. Don't judge your intake by someone else. We are not all alike. Eat and drink less — join that wonderful organization the Weight Watchers and learn to balance intake. Don't try to take weight off by exercise — it can't be done. To take off one pound it is necessary for the average person to walk fifty miles, and this could make you rather sore and very hungry. The less you eat, the better you feel — *try it!*

7

WHAT CAN MASSAGE DO?

Massage is one of the oldest forms of medicine and before the advent of modern drugs it was used all over the world. One of the first great physicians, Hippocrates *c*. 460 - *c*. 380 B.C., often called the father of medicine, is reported as saying — "The physician must be experienced in many things, but assuredly in rubbing." Rubbing can bind a joint that is too loose or loosen a joint that is too tight.

In India and ancient Greece the groom always rubbed his horse down with his naked hands and this ensured that the steed had a much finer coat than the English horse which was groomed with a brush and curry comb. In 1825 John Grosvenor, a surgeon, used massage friction in his practice, and his skill and reputation became great. He was particularly re-nowned for his cures of stiff joints and lameness.

In 1870, Dr N.B. Emerson gave a most interesting description of the treatment of lomi-lomi practised in the Sandwich Isles. This was a healthful form of relaxing passive motion which the Hawaiians bestow upon each other as an act of kindness and their act of hospitality to a visitor. When footsore and weary, when no position affords rest, so that sleep appears impossible it relieves soreness, stiffness and lameness and soothes the person to sleep so that excessive exercise is not felt the next day, but a lovely suppleness of muscle and ease of joint is procured. The Hawaiians have a great appreciation of the physical wants of the tired system which Dr Emerson thinks would be as well for other civilized nations to copy. They have many ways of administering the lomi-lomi. The patient lies down on a mat, and the operator, who is usually old and experienced, begins rubbing, squeezing, kneading and stretching all the muscles. They often swim long distances, and when exhausted are revived by the lomi-lomi. The chiefs appear to have wonderful physiques, and naturally they are the ones who get the most treatment.

Whilst I was doing a little R.A.F. service, last war, in South-East Asia, I was fortunate to make friends with a Cassi tribesman who taught me a few things. Many years ago these people were head-hunters, but now they excel at flighting arrows at tiny bamboo targets. They even shoot birds in flight, and fish in the river, but to go with them on a wild boar hunt is certainly an alarming experience. As the boar madly charges they stand their ground, wait until they can see the redness in their eyes, then swish, swish, swish, three arrows in quick succession, the last one only when the maddened boar is feet away.

However, the feat that intrigued me most was when the young men carried a large wicker basket on their backs, with a strap round their foreheads, and ran up a very steep hill, whilst carrying a passenger in the basket. These young men had enormous calf muscles, and my attention was drawn to the method of leg massage. As soon as one man had put down his passenger one of the rested athletes would massage his friend for a long period, not with his hands, but massaging with his feet, and this was most skilfully done. Despite the terrific strain of this running climb their legs were beautifully supple and their naked feet as perfect as nature.

Back to Britain where massage is slowly losing favour with many hospitals, I well remember tests we did at the Westwood Health and Strength Club many years ago. When a boy had done a series of feats of endurance or strength to his limit, we gave him a short, sharp session of massage on the muscles involved, and he could then improve on his previous performance. How can we neglect this therapeutic science to improve not only the athlete, but also more important, the sufferer? It is a wonderful science, and if care is used it can only do good.

Don't massage over varicose veins, or any part that is inflamed, or over broken skin. If in doubt, consult your doctor, and always remember that after massage we must move all the joints to their fullest extent. Today in hospitals the physiotherapy departments treat many patients with various machines, but very rarely do they use the finest machine of all, the HAND. Massage is a very old science, and years ago it was only performed with the hands. Today the hand appears to have lost favour, but I am certain that there is no substitute for the skilled hand. In most cases the hand can do far more than the machine, and even during diagnosis, the hand is the first essential. It is possible for most people to learn to give themselves hand massage, and this is one of my reasons for writing this book.

As you progress you will find the hand and fingers getting more supple and stronger, and as the skill improves you can use more pressure, but never use it to the point of hurting the tissues. There are many scientific names in massage, but I propose to omit most, and keep this book mainly for the suffering layman. Before I give my understanding of massage and movement we have many cases to study, and I hope you will bear with me if I leave your massage instructions until later.

Just as there are many different types of people, there are various types of arthritis, and whilst it is not necessary to go into fine detail, there is one unusual type that I must include — CLIMACTERIC ARTHRITIS. This is a kind of rheumatoid arthritis, and affects mostly the small joints of ladies at or about the change of life. It is certainly associated with the cessation of menstruation, and is it not possible that the former menstrual flow helped to clear toxic and acid wastes from the body? Once this stops, there could be a build up in the system, and we are aware that there is a disturbance of the endocrine functions. Often the patient is suffering from low vitality, nervous debility, and depression. I have had patients who were unable to fasten a button, and were afraid they were going to be crippled for life. It is necessary to reassure these ladies that as the glands settle down the arthritis will start to improve, and in most cases a perfect recovery will occur when the menopause is over, provided that they keep mobile and cheerful. Having the knowledge that this is so I am very upset when a patient submits to surgery at this time of bodily change. Please give nature a chance and help by adjusting mentally and physically.

Contact your doctor for a medical check, there are things that can help, particularly if you are anaemic, which is pretty often at this period.

8

STIMULATION AND DRUGS

The body has a wonderful inbuilt mechanism to protect the heart, and prevent one from damaging the body by extreme exertion. When an athlete is pushed to his, or her, physical limit, and then endeavours to carry on, a chemical change occurs in the bloodstream and the muscles go into a violent cramp so that further movement is not possible. This is nature's way of saving the body from permanent damage. If an athlete had been taking drugs, (many do) to improve his performance, he has upset the natural balance, and the body's reaction is delayed, sometimes with grim results.

Britain's wonderful cyclist Tommy Simpson was so keen to win the Tour de France that he took stimulants, and despite falling off his bicycle three times, when exhausted, he remounted and then died. Without drugs he would not have been able to mount the second time, but the stimulant destroyed his natural inbuilt protection.

Another rule of the body is that every period of stimulation is followed by a corresponding period of *depression*. In other words, if you stimulate the body above normal it will certainly drop below that later. Whilst there is a rhythm in the body, nature tries to keep us on an even keel, but here comes trouble. With drug stimulation and many pop stars take stimulants to pep themselves up for a performance, the following depression often makes these people do things which are foreign to their nature, and sometimes they even make violent mistakes.

We have done those things which we ought not to have done and there is *no health* in us. Whilst every period of stimulation is always followed by a period of depression the opposite is not so. Each period of depression is not followed by a period of stimulation, and what often happens is that the depressed patient is given tablets for his depression. These so often upset his nervous system that he just doesn't know what ails him. I often wonder if, when people do the most absurd things, they are suffering from double depression.

Further to this short discussion on drugs please remember that health is to be won, not by a bottle of medicine, but by A WAY OF LIVING. If drugs could make health, doctors and chemists would be at the top of the health list, but I am sorry to say that they are almost at the bottom.

9

EATING

To a great extent, we are what we eat, but no two people are alike, and what suits one does not necessarily suit another. By the age of thirty man should understand his body, and know what suits him best. Don't be like the rather stout lady who came to my surgery one morning and said, "I feel terrible this morning — but then I always do when I have had bananas for breakfast." For heaven's sake, and your health's sake, if a food does not agree with you, CAST IT OUT.

To illustrate a difference in people, I discovered that I was far fitter, and certainly able to work harder, without breakfast. Since then I have not eaten breakfast, except a few times on holiday, for forty-five years. Please don't get me wrong. I am not suggesting that you do the same, but to me it is amazing that so many medical men insist that it is essential to eat a good breakfast to get one to work, and complete the morning. Let us now examine this strange statement.

When we eat a meal it is many hours before the food passes through the stomach. Only then can it travel through the long tubes of intestines and more hours pass before it is assimilated into the bloodstream, and only then can it give any nourishment to the body. So how is it that one should have breakfast to endure the morning's work? Surely it is with yesterday's food that we are sustained today.

Another vital point is that one should only eat when hungry, and eating breakfast or any other meal when there is no hunger is not good health sense. Something more to study is that after sleeping all night, is it not possible that we have not earned a meal? Wild animals and ancient peoples hunted their food and thereby built up an appetite first. However, as I said before, no two people are alike, and if you are genuinely hungry at breakfast time, eat some.

A word of warning to people who have no morning appetite, do not think that by listening to the experts you should reluctantly eat some food to preserve your strength. It will only take away your strength in the process of trying to digest unwanted food. Another mistake is eating a tiny breakfast. Once food is eaten the gastric juices begin to flow, and they don't know that you are only having half a slice of toast. They are stimulated by the first bite and flow for a full meal. They tend to get annoyed at having only a little food and have been known to try to digest the stomach walls. It must be a proper meal or no food, or the acid gastric juice will be left in the stomach to cause trouble, but again so much depends on the individual and you should be the final judge.

I think you can regulate your own diet, but there are some foods which are really detrimental to rheumatism. In my experience these are rhubarb and strawberries, and some people react badly to oranges, but all fried foods and pies, pasties, cream, cakes, chocolates and sweets are acid forming. In the citrus fruits, oranges, apples, pears, lemons, grapefruits and lime, it is not good to eat any of these with bread. This is an incompatible mixture where the acid in the fruits fights with the starch in the bread. The ideal is to eat citrus fruits alone, as then they tend to change easily in the digestion and form alkaline in the bloodstream, and to be healthy it is necessary that the blood is slightly alkaline.

Each day try to eat some fresh fruit and salad. The foods which have life in them are best eaten fresh and raw. Live foods make us more lively and healthier. This means food as it comes out of the ground or from the tree, such as grated raw carrot, cauliflower, cabbage, celery, mint, watercress, and besides the citrus fruits figs, prunes, dates and raisins. Heavy red meat should be eaten sparingly. Use lamb, tripe, cheese, and fowl for your protein, but always remember that one food suits one person but doesn't suit another.

I remember meeting a learned professor of dietetics, who displayed huge double chins, and what looked like a large brewer's goitre below his ample chest. Most people think that a pain or gnawing in the stomach is a sign of hunger, when, in fact, it is often an irritation suffered by a sour stomach carrying acid residue from the last meal that had not been perfectly digested. This is the time to miss a meal and drink water to disperse the acid and cleanse the stomach.

Please don't think you will pass on by missing a meal or two. This is the finest way to improve the health, rest the overworked stomach, and ease the pain. When we deprive the body of food the wonderful power that controls the life force starts to live on its reserves of fats, sugars, and even on the system's waste material which is in everyone's body. There is no danger whatever unless the fast is carried on for a long time. In fact there is a wonderful improvement to be gained in health from short, periodic fasts, and as the body then lives on its reserves and fat we can say it is using up its own badness.

I was 14 years old when I first fasted, and my rheumatism improved at once, but I confess I rather overdid it, and having only 14 years of badness in my poor body, I nearly starved after having nothing but water for seven days. Since then I have fasted at least once each year, and proved to my satisfaction that it is the greatest of all medicines. Please don't attempt a long fast until you know a great deal more about it, but how about trying a one-day fast right now? There is only one correct way to do a one-day fast, and it takes three days.

1st DAY — Reduce all meals by fifty per cent. Cut out tea, coffee, alcohol and smoking.

2nd DAY — No food of any kind, but take a glass of water as often as possible· whilst the stomach is empty the water helps to wash it inside.

3rd DAY — Start with a very small meal. I suggest one slice of brown toast, with one poached egg and half a glass of warm milk. If you suffer from catarrh or chest trouble, omit the milk. It is a perfect food for a calf but in humans it can upset the sinuses, chest, and asthmatic conditions. Try not to eat for at least 4 hours after the first meal and keep the rest of the day's meals to fifty per cent of your usual intake.

After your first fast, make a fresh start, and eat less, choosing your food more carefully, omitting all foods that do not agree with you, eating slower, and chewing the food until it goes down in a liquid state.

10

DRUG PROMOTIONS

We have tended to rely on our doctors who are so often overworked, and it is now time to do a little for ourselves. Recently a G.P. reported that he got 100,000 words of drug information each month. He said, "I have a choice, either to ignore new drugs, and possibly deny my patients access to potentially life-saving treatment, such as the beta-blockers, or I launch out with prescriptions of drugs unheard of in my student days."

As drugs become more powerful their potential for poisonous side effects increases. How soon is it before attendance at the doctor's surgery brings greater hazards from treatment than from the original conflict? Figures from America,* published in the *New York Times* show that about half the non-fatal complications of surgery may be preventable and that adverse drug reactions kill 10,000 people annually. Drug permutations damage 300,000 and the injudicious use of antibiotics may account for 100,000 deaths each year. Over fifty new drugs are presented in Britain each year, and approximately forty-eight million pounds is spent on drug promotions.

*Oldham Evening Chronicle, 9/2/77.

In 1967 English surgeon Arthur Dickenson Wright, aged 69, attacked the over-use of antibiotics and claimed that twenty million pounds each year could be saved if the number of prescriptions was reduced to what was really necessary. He also added that probably 10,000 people in this country were permanently drunk because they were overdosed with streptomycin. Surely it is time that we examined modern medicine very carefully. Medicine claims to be scientific, but science demands exactitude.

Just one little item of everyday medication will prove that there is nothing exact in medicine. A girl of, say six stones is often given the same amount of an injection as a man of fifteen stones. When we realize that the man has almost twice the volume of blood as the girl we cannot really call this scientific; and the same is true of tablets. In fact this is often the cause of greater side effects — and what about the big difference in the age of patients which is seldom taken into account?

One of my patients once experimented after being given a new drug to help his breathing. He was told to take three tablets each day. After the first early morning tablet the breathing was much easier, but the patient started to shake violently — quite unable to even hold a cup of tea. He took no more tablets that day but tried half a tablet the next morning with the same result. The following morning he tried a quarter of a tablet and he was still shaking. After further trials it was found that one eighth of a tablet per day was satisfactory. His breathing was easy and he was not shaking. This was one twenty-fourth of the prescribed dose. I know he should have gone back to the doctors, but what if he had persevered with the full dose?

You may now say what has this to do with rheumatism? There are some hundreds of drugs for rheumatism and many have side effects, so if you are troubled that way, get back to your doctor before any harm is done.

11

SUPPORTS

In recent years there has been a vast increase in body supports of all descriptions. Every day one can see the poor neck sufferers walking about with stiffly held heads supported by a thick neck collar. Whilst it is imperative that a broken limb must be supported, these people do not have broken necks. Why the collar? It is once again the strange idea that rest makes for cure. Rest makes for weakness and the muscles which are not used deteriorate rapidly, and it takes a great deal of exercise and a long time to rebuild them. Rest is helpful in the very early stages of extreme pain, but I have known people to wear a neck collar for years, with the result that all the neck muscles have wasted, the bursa have stopped secreting and arthritis has completely locked every cervical vertebra.

This also applies to lumbar supports and the quickest way to weaken the lower back is to encase it in plaster. I am certainly of the opinion that 90% of these supports are unnecessary and very often detrimental. I usually tell patients that I cannot treat them unless they agree to dispense with their support and become mobile.

One man who came to me wearing a huge neck collar agreed to stop wearing it any longer, but insisted that he must keep it so that when he had to see the specialist in three months' time at the hospital, he could put it on for the said appointment. After three months' treatment and full neck exercises, he reported to the hospital, put the unused collar on outside, and was examined by the same specialist who had examined him three months before. The specialist said: "That collar has cured you. You have no need to wear it any longer." The poor man never explained. How long will it be before the medical profession discovers that without movement any part of the body deteriorates, and even joints that already have some arthritis in them can be improved by intensive movement?

I have had the privilege of meeting many wonderful people who were badly handicapped, and one I shall never forget was Mr Arthur Lees, M.B.E., one of the originators of the Inskip League of Friends for the Disabled, 1949, and as the Honorary Secretary he spent many hours standing typing correspondence when it was not possible for him to sit. Pain never stopped him, and he could only get around in his three-wheeled invacar due to his massive spondylitis — the whole of his spine was completely locked and immovable. Most people would have stayed put, but not Arthur, who worked like a beaver for the League and was later honoured with the M.B.E. by the Queen.

In his early twenties he started to have back pains, and was put into a large plaster cast from his neck to his hips for four years during which time each vertebra grew into the next with complete loss of movement, and then this terrible arthritis spread to his hips and knees. We managed to keep movement in his ankles and feet so that with two sticks he could just negotiate low steps.

At fifty years of age, Arthur was killed by a heavy lorry whilst on a trip to Blackpool in his invacar. His tragic death was a terrible blow both to his grand wife and to the Inskip League, but the great work he started goes on.

12

POSTURE

We have touched somewhat on diet, and on some of the causes of rheumatism, but now we will examine posture and movement which is vital for health. Since the advent of the motor car and later the television many people do not move enough, and by sitting too much often adapt to a very bad posture. Test yourself in the standing position and find the curves of the spine — Fig. 3. The spine has great strength and flexibility, but the character of motion and the relationship between two vertebrae is of great importance, because any slight deviation of one vertebra may lead to disruption of the whole spine. The spine can be a great deal of trouble if it is out of line in any part, and because the spinal cord is enclosed until the nerves branch out from each side of every vertebra, any alteration in the spine can cause pressure on these nerves and pain is felt along any part or all of the nerve in question. Even pain in a big toe can originate in the nerve situated in the lower back. This is an example where it would be useless massaging the big toe when the cause is in the back.

As most people know, each vertebra is separated from its fellow by a tough, unique piece of cartilage called a vertebral disc. A most well-known condition of

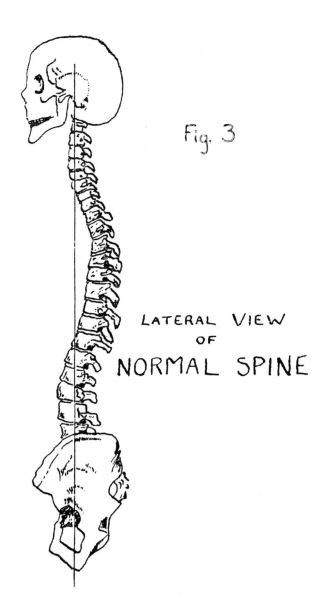

Fig. 3

LATERAL VIEW
OF
NORMAL SPINE

the spine is the slipped disc. I have been amazed at the number of slipped discs which were diagnosed when the patients were suffering from some other back condition. Like pop music and other happenings which originated in the States, the slipped disc has become fashionable here.

A surgeon in New York said: "Eighty per cent of slipped disc patients sent to me for the operation had no sign of this when opened." I wonder if the patient was told, and whether he received a monetary rebate or discount?

Most spinal troubles are caused as the result of bad posture and incorrect lifting. If you suffer from low back pain, sciatica, pain in the shoulders, arm or leg, or even in the fingers or toes, it could be due to pressure on the spinal nerves, adhesions, stiffness of the spine, tension of the spinal muscles, or curvature of the spine itself, but the most likely source of the trouble is FLATTENED DISCS, not slipped discs, Fig. 4.

Fig 4

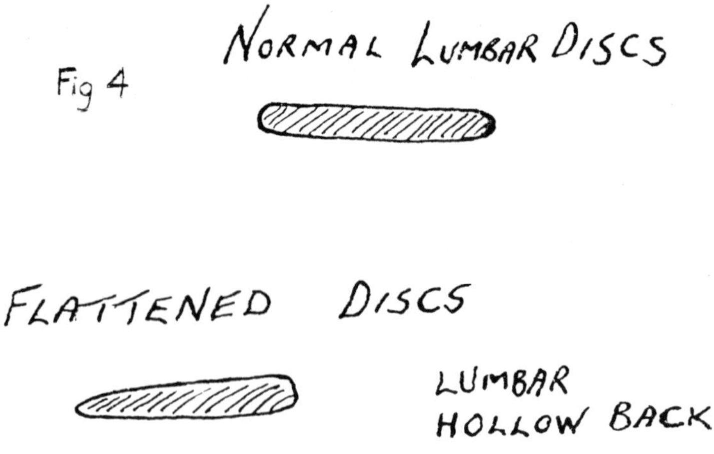

NORMAL LUMBAR DISCS

FLATTENED DISCS

LUMBAR HOLLOW BACK

Let us now examine discs, without being too technical. The discs separate the vertebrae from each other and keep the spinal nerves free, providing a strong, smooth elastic cushion to enable easy spinal movements. The spine is curved to give greater strength and flexibility than it would do if it were straight. Pressure is more or less fairly evenly distributed centrally on the discs, which have a nucleus of water but if there is too much curve in one part of the spine the pressure becomes displaced, and just as a stiletto heel takes the weight of the body on one tiny point, vastly increasing the pounds per square inch, so does the weight increase on one part of the disc, resulting in the *Flattened Disc*.

Calculations have been made which suggest that a twelve stone man can exert over a quarter of a ton of pressure on his discs. Take an exaggerated forward curve in the lumbar spine and compare it with the straight spine (Fig. 5). It is easy to see that the weight is concentrated towards the back of the disc, and this is flattening the disc, making it wedge-shaped (Fig. 5a). This puts a terrific strain on the back of the disc and allows the posterior process of the adjoining vertebrae to become too close to each other, trapping the soft tissues between, causing inflammation and pain. In extreme cases pressure becomes centred on to the spinal nerve where it emerges from the cord, and this can cause trouble all the way down this nerve.

Sciatica is a painful nerve condition, sometimes travelling from the lower back to the toes, and mostly caused by pressure on nerves in the lower back. In the upper back we often have too much backward curve which throws weight and strain on the front of the discs, resulting in a flattened disc, wedge-shaped with

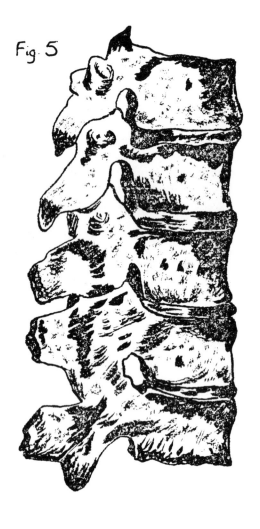

Fig. 5

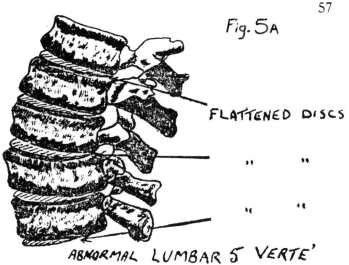

Fig. 5A

FLATTENED DISCS

" "

" "

ABNORMAL LUMBAR 5 VERTE'

the narrow flat part to the front (Fig. 6). There is not so much weight bearing on these dorsal discs as there is on the lumbar ones, but often we have too much curve backwards in the upper back, and too much forward curve in the lower, as the body is striving to get into a reasonable centre of gravity (Fig. 7) and this is one reason for general all-over backache. The whole body tires due to the uneven strain on all the back muscles. This condition calls for corrective exercise, not for tablets.

The spine has a tremendous task to perform, and if the posture is bad the strain is far greater, which can be the beginning of arthritis. Good posture means that the body weight is transmitted through the skeleton, from bone to bone, with little strain on ligaments and minimum demands on muscles. This is equally important in sitting or standing. A sagging posture

KYPHOSIS (THORACIC CURVE)

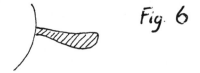

Fig. 6

KYPHO LORDOSIS

Fig. 7

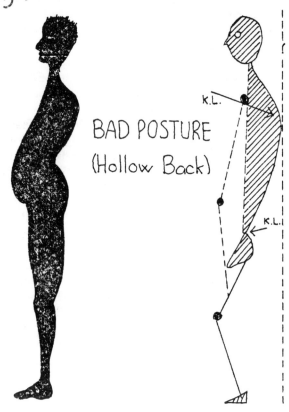

BAD POSTURE
(Hollow Back)

K.L.

K.L.

with an increase in the spinal curves is detrimental but if the patient can move the spine, exercise can cure this condition.

Study the two sketches, then look into a full-length mirror while you are standing in your usual posture. Then stand with your back to the wall and your heels 3 inches away. Can you put your hand between the wall and your lower back? If so your lumbar curve is too great and you require special exercise.

Does your upper back curve too far posterially? Does your head poke forward? Are you more like Fig. 9 than Fig. 8? A hollow low back is often seen in ladies who have had heavy babies, and have never been taught how to bend up afterwards. I well remember a patient coming to see me from Southern Ireland. She had a most ghastly hollow back and I immediately said: "You have had very heavy babies."

"No," she replied, "the heaviest child I ever had was six pounds," but on further questioning she admitted that she had triplets. She was in great pain, but one treatment and six months of one specific exercise cured her completely.

In sciatica and low back pain I find that four people out of ten have hollow backs. Now for trouble. In almost every hospital physiotherapy department these four people are grouped with six more or less straight-backed people, and all are given the same exercises, the most prominent one being: lying face downwards, lifting the head and chest, and many times lifting the legs off the floor to hollow the back and stretch the stomach muscles. This is a good exercise for straight-backed people but a tragedy for those with hollow backs (Fig. 10).

Many years ago I protested strongly to an

60

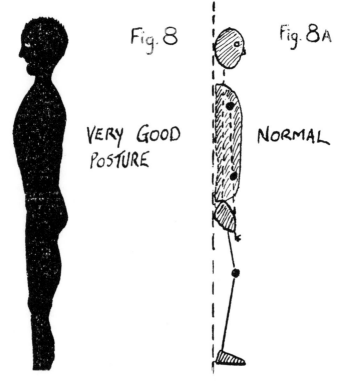

Fig. 8

Fig. 8A

VERY GOOD
POSTURE

NORMAL

orthopaedic surgeon about the folly of this exercise for
people with hollow backs, and demonstrated my
special exercise to cure these suffering people, but
whilst he fully agreed, nothing was done, doubtless
because I was not a medically qualified man. I intend
to show you this one exercise and urge all people with
hollow backs to get down to bending the *RIGHT* way
— just the opposite to the medical way.

The apparatus required is one stool about nine
inches high or the bottom stair at home. Sit on the

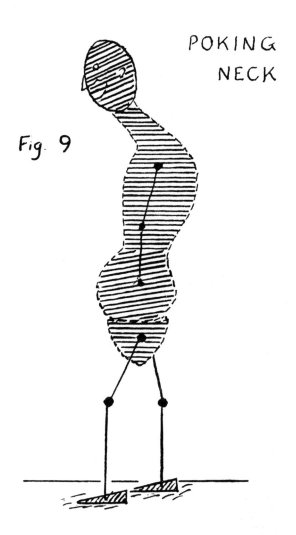

POKING NECK

Fig. 9

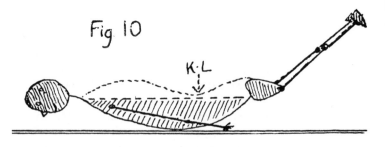

Fig 10

K·L

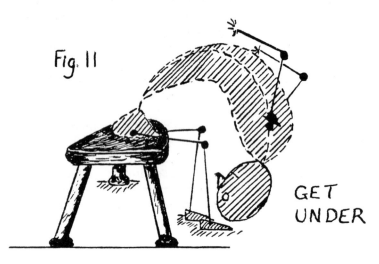

Fig. 11

GET
UNDER

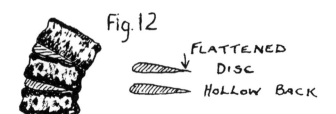

Fig. 12

FLATTENED
DISC

HOLLOW BACK

stool with your legs open as wide as possible with your feet firmly on the floor in front and to the side of the stool. Put your hands behind your neck with your elbows pointing forwards. Every effort is now made to curl the back by pushing out the hollow and trying to get the head between the knees with the back as rounded as possible. Once down, start to bounce by lifting the back upwards about ten inches (no more) then bouncing down between the knees using the weight of the upper body and trying to get lower and lower. Do not come to the upright position until this is finished. It is not necessary to use strength but rather a smooth rhythm and the bounce should almost lift the buttocks off the stool whilst you roll into a tight ball. That stretches the muscles, tendons and ligaments of the lower back, Fig. 11.

Start with eight bounces and gradually increase the number as you become more supple to a possible fifty. Many hundreds of my patients have cured their low back troubles with this one exercise. It isn't easy. It hurts and takes time, but if you persevere, you will be rewarded for your efforts. From now on you must not bend backwards at any time. Even painting a ceiling is bad.

Try to learn a different stance from your former posture. When standing, lean just a little forward, taking the weight off your heels and putting your centre of gravity more towards the toes. This takes the strain off the hollow back. Don't wear house slippers or shoes with very low heels.

Why does this one exercise produce such good results? Again we go to those discs. With the hollow back we find that the discs are flattened and wedge-shaped with the thin part on the outside (Fig.

12), and as we take the curve out of the hollow and straighten up the discs return to a better shape due to the pressure at the extreme edge being relieved, and once this is accomplished the water content in the disc helps to even out its shape.

The vertebrae of the spine are bound together by very strong tendons, ligaments, and muscles, all of which will stretch even in late middle age. Please get stretching. Hollow backs are the most painful, but if your back is straight and painful, then the opposite exercise is for you. Bend backwards and wear low heels. I appreciate that there are other causes of back pain. If in doubt consult your doctor. The upper back does not give quite the same amount of trouble but so many people are developing round shoulders that I must include a very good exercise for this condition.
BYRAM'S DOORWAY STRETCH. Stand with feet apart about eight inches from any inside open door, and placing the forearms and hands on each side of the door frame lean through the doorway as far as possible keeping the body still. Don't stick the tummy out (Fig. 13). This exercise opens the chest by stretching the pectoral muscles, and contracts the upper back. It also helps to take the strain off the dorsal discs, which are often flattened at the front. This is an excellent exercise which not only improves the back, but loosens the shoulders and helps breathing. It is not strenuous and one only need do it once or twice each day with around six repetitions.

Many people have been treated for disc lesions by traction in hospital, and in theory this should do an immense amount of good by opening the vertebrae and taking the strain off the discs and spinal nerves, but the results are often disappointing. My explanation

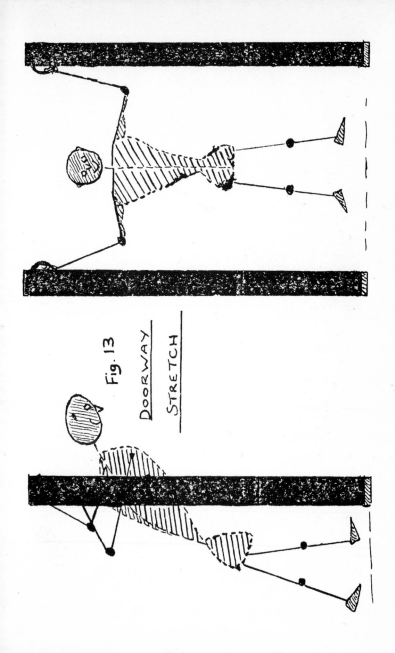

Fig. 13

DOORWAY STRETCH

Photo 1 — see page 101

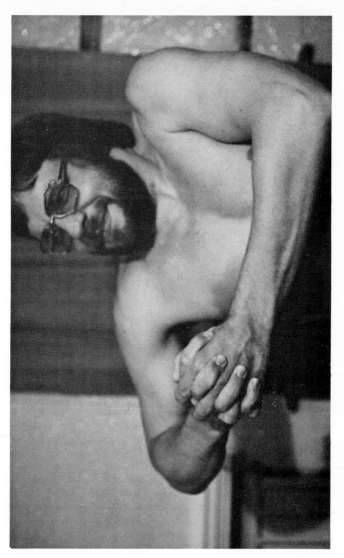

Photo 2 — see page 102

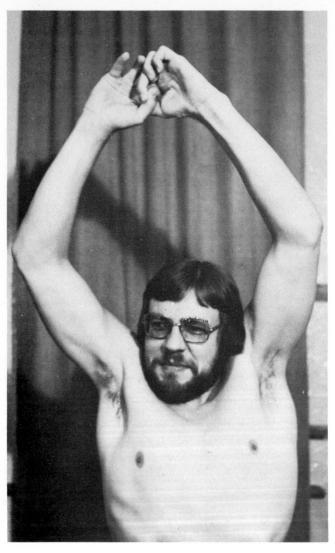

Photo 3 – see page 102

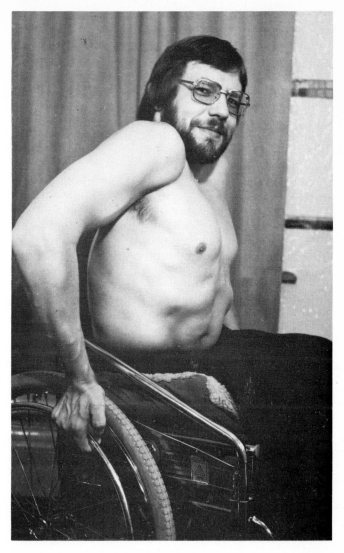

Photo 4 – see page 102

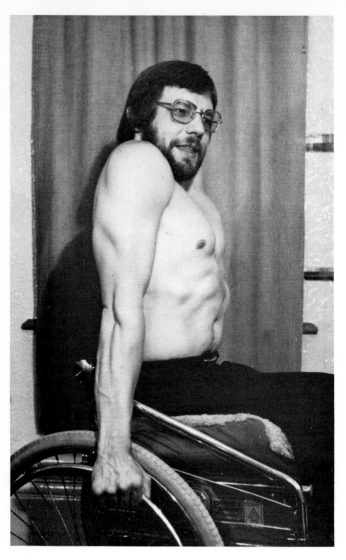

Photo 5 — see page 103

Photo 6 – see page 104

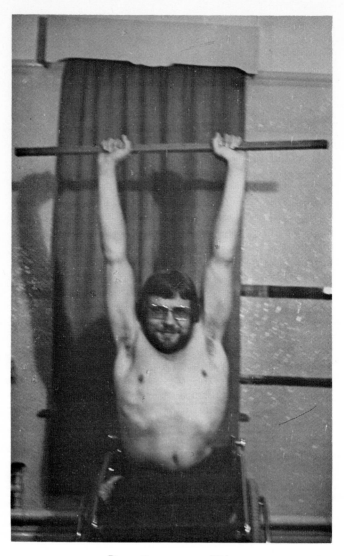

Photo 7 – see page 104

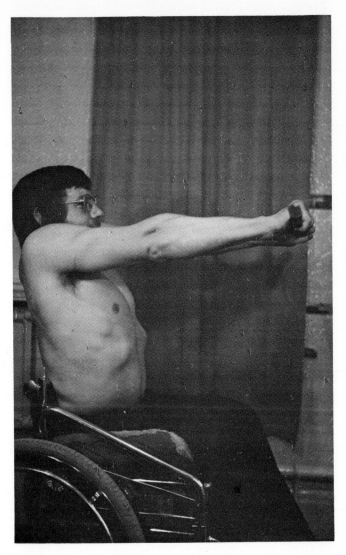

Photo 8 – see page 104

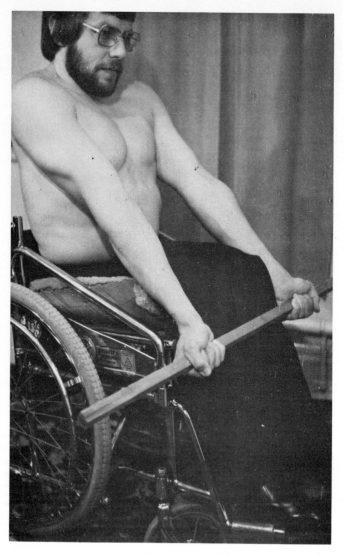

Photo 9 – see page 104

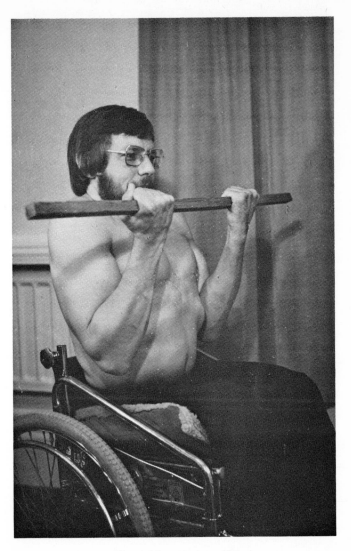

Photo 10 – see page 104

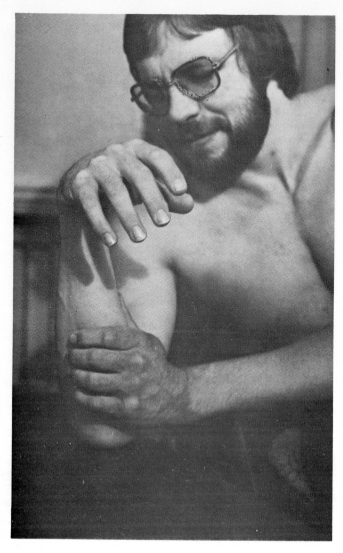

Photo 11 — see page 106

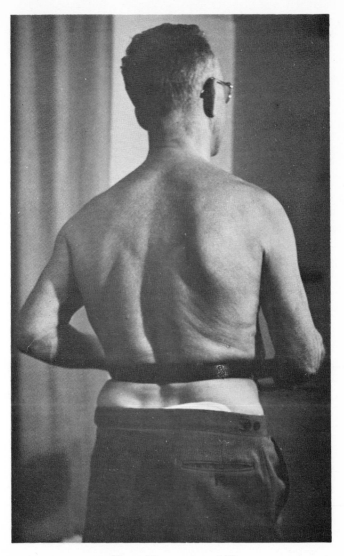

Photo 12 – see page 113

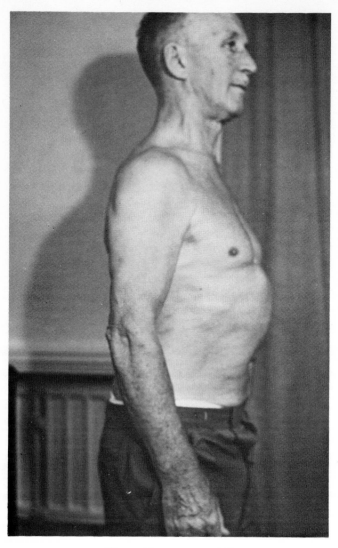

Photo 13 — see page 128

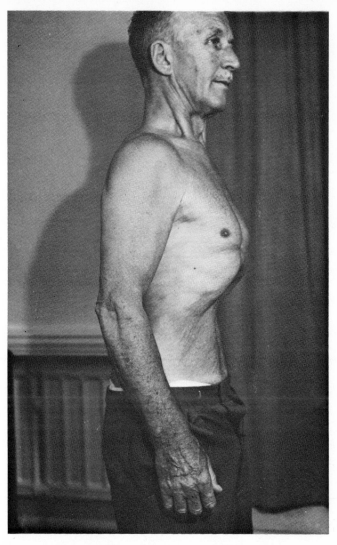

Photo 14 – see page 128

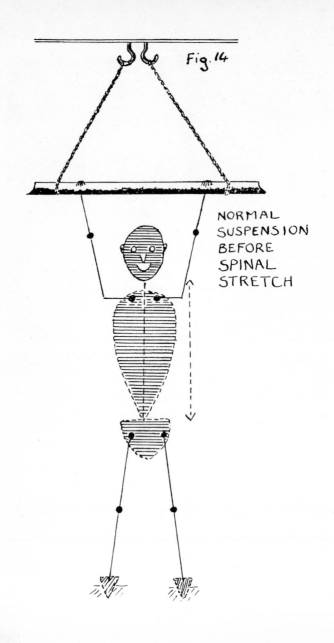

Fig. 14

NORMAL
SUSPENSION
BEFORE
SPINAL
STRETCH

is that it is very hard for people in pain to relax, and as the pressure of the traction increases, the muscles of the back become more and more tense, thus a tug of war which fails to open the spine, and tires the tightened spinal muscles.

Here is an exercise that relies on the patient, and in my opinion is second to none for stretching the spine, improving flattened discs, and taking pressure off spinal nerves. The apparatus required is two pieces of string, two small hooks, and one piece of wood, four feet long and one inch round. You could use any round stick for this excellent exercise. Fix the hooks two inches apart in a convenient place in the ceiling (the bathroom is perhaps best). Fit the two pieces of string to each hook, then fasten the other ends to the wood, so that it is level at the height you can reach it easily with the feet flat on the ground (Fig. 14). The exercise demands that at no time must the string become too tight. Holding the wood with both hands a little wider than the width of your shoulders, proceed to turn the body by shuffling the feet round slowly and at the same time stretching the arms and body to ensure that the string is never tight. At each quarter turn pause for a couple of seconds then concentrate on lifting the chest and the spine. As you turn, the twist of the strings lifts the stick higher and you are lifting and stretching all the spine to keep the string slack. Keep your heels flat on the floor, stretch your arms, lift your shoulders, lift your chest and spine, and concentrate on getting taller.

If you will do this wonderful exercise for one minute twice daily, not only will you feel taller and fitter, but very often your disc troubles will vanish and your posture improvement will be far greater than you

E

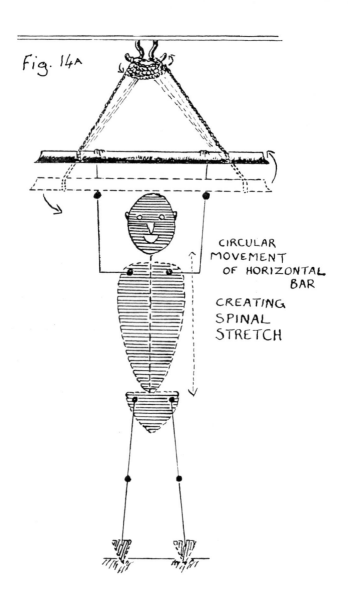

Fig. 14ᴬ

CIRCULAR
MOVEMENT
OF HORIZONTAL
BAR

CREATING
SPINAL
STRETCH

could ever imagine was possible.

This exercise is also particularly good for scoliosis of the spine. Scoliosis is a sideways bend in the spine, usually in the upper region but sometimes in the lower, and often in both, when we can have a bend to the left in the lower with a bend to the right in the upper part. (Fig. 15). In an upper bend to the left a good exercise is to put the right arm over the head, grasp the left ear, take a deep breath, hold it, and then quickly lean the upper body over to the left as far as possible (Fig. 16). As you bend, the right side, which has been contracted is extended, and holding the full breath lifts, and opens the ribs on the right.

Still with the spine, which is wonderful, let us take a brief look at a part that often gives pain and plenty of trouble — the SACRO-ILIAC joints. In my effort to keep this book non-technical I find this joint a little difficult to explain. The human spine sustains the weight of the upper body, and this is mainly transmitted through the sacrum and the ilium (pelvis) to the legs via the hips; thus we have the sacro-iliac joints supporting the weight of the trunk. These two joints are held by very strong ligaments, but sudden, abnormal or unreasonable stress can stretch these ligaments so that they relax their hold on the large bones, then the joint moves a little, and the result is a very painful sacro-iliac strain. Mostly this is caused by twisting the body whilst lifting a heavy object. When lifting always bend the knees fully, and face the object without twisting.

We often find that when the sacro-iliac joint has been strained it is possible to disturb it even by reaching over the front seat of the car to pick up a light brief-case from the back seat, as it is the twist that

SCOLIOSIS
WITH
OPPOSITE
BEND IN
LUMBAR
SPINE

Fig. 15

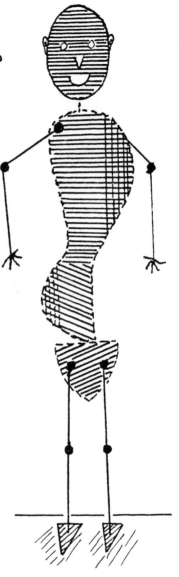

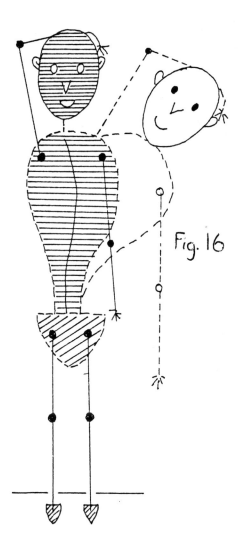

Fig. 16

causes the trouble and if one can always avoid twisting by keeping in a forward plane, even a weak joint will recover. Many causes of sciatica are caused by pressures on the nerves around the sacro-iliac joint. If the pain is not too great I can help you to manipulate this joint, but if the pain is severe, get the doctor, or better still, an osteopath.

The self help is first a really good soak in a hot soapy bath with the addition of four tablespoons of olive oil, well mixed. When wet, hot, and fully relaxed sit over the outer edge of the bath, one leg out and one inside, as if riding a narrow horse. Put your hands behind your neck, then twist the body around quickly but smoothly, rotating first to the right and then to the left a few times whilst gripping the sides of the bath with your thigh and knees to steady the pelvis and confine the movement to the lower back. Often you will hear a fairly loud click and then feel a good deal of relief.

The sacro-iliac joint strain is the most common, but we must look at other strains of the lower back. There are two — the lumbo-sacral strain and the strain of the fourth and fifth lower vertebrae. In both of these, the pelvis is rotated a little, causing one side to be somewhat in front of the other, and one hip to be more prominent than its fellow (Fig. 17). This can also occur in the sacro-iliac strain, and in rare cases in all three, or a combination of any two. Here is your helpful self-manipulation using the bar and string but stopping short of the full lift. In this position endeavour to do a short hula-hula movement to the side that doesn't stand out. Keeping the feet together and the string slack, sway away from the bad prominent side and then back, trying not to go beyond the centre line (Fig. 18).

LUMBAR SCOLIOSIS

Fig. 17

WITH
RIGHT HIP
PROMINENT

Push

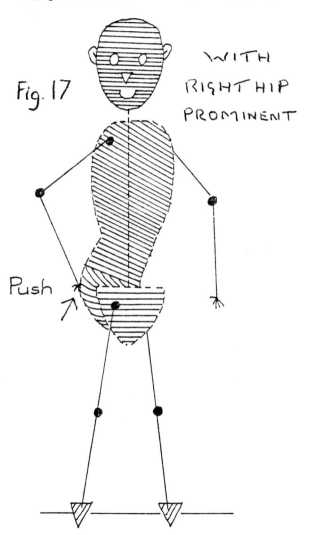

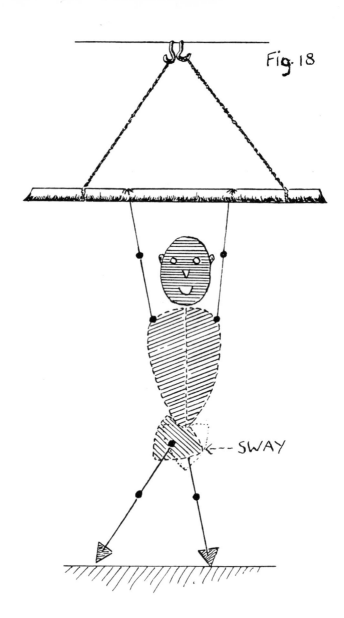

Fig. 18

SWAY

After this exercise if the bad side is still prominent, a further exercise is to be done daily. If it is the right hip, stand with your feet apart, and your right hand on your right hip. Push hard, and sway to the left (Fig. 19) again trying not to pass the centre as you come back from the left sway.

In many cases of low back trouble the sciatic nerve is involved, and this can produce severe pain all down the course of the nerve even to the toes. As the inflammation increases the nerve shortens, and tends to kink almost like an old electric wire. A quick but painful remedy is to stretch the nerve vigorously by standing in front of a chair with the foot of the painful leg resting on the chair. Straighten both legs, pull the toes and foot of the bad leg towards you, (this stretches the sciatic nerve), put both hands behind your neck and then very quickly bend the trunk as far forwards as possible, keeping both knees straight and stiff. This must be done only once, the principal effect is to give one vigorous stretch to the shortened sciatic nerve (Fig. 20)

Here is just one more exercise, this time for the knee. Many times early arthritis starts in the knee, usually under the patella, and if the cap is not free to move it is not possible to bend the leg fully; neither is it wise to try to bend the leg until the patella* is fully free. To loosen the patella, sit on a bed or on the floor with your legs straight, place a small cushion under the knee, and try to move the kneecap with your thumb and finger, first sideways, then up and down. This is not easy at first and you may have to adjust the cushion until the leg is fully relaxed when it should be possible to mobilize the cap (Fig. 21).

*The patella is the kneecap.

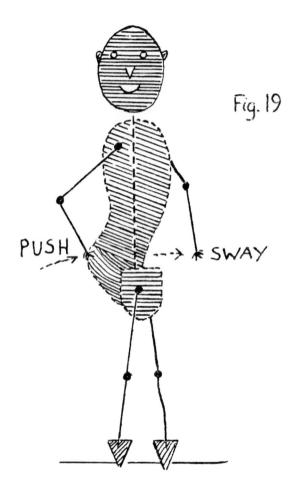

Fig. 19

PUSH

SWAY

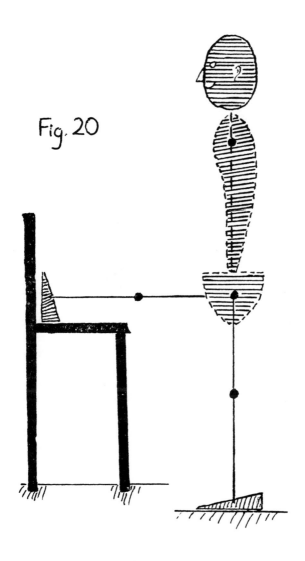

Fig. 20

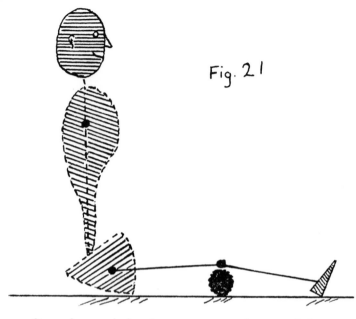

Fig. 21

Once the cap is freed you can move it up and down
by tightening your thigh muscles. Relax between each
movement and watch the patella fall down loosely.
With a fair degree of practise it is possible to flick the
kneecap at least fifty times per minute. This becomes a
type of muscle control, and it is advisable to do one
thousand flicks each day. It takes little energy and with
practise can be done standing. To make it harder
place the palm of one hand over the patella, pressing
gently towards the toes. Now flick against this
resistance — an excellent exercise (Fig. 21).

13

HEAT

In the last chapter we did a few specific exercises for rheumatic pains and strains. We can now examine the necessity for keeping the body warm. It is most important that the body temperature is stable at around 98°, but circumstances can alter this, with detrimental effects, particularly to the rheumatic sufferer. Warmth comes from inside you, and the person with a good circulation can usually keep warm with exercises. A quick walk of a couple of miles stimulates the circulation and this warmth lasts a long time. The body heat from sitting in front of a fire vanishes as soon as one moves away.

For the people who are unable to exercise it is essential that they are always warmly clad, and there is room here for a little knowledge. Firstly nylon and terylene underwear are not good. These materials cannot 'breathe'. They don't absorb perspiration, and they become cold and clammy even on a warm day. For rheumatism wool is best next to the skin, cotton is next best, and then silk (if you can afford it). On the market there is now special underwear made for rheumatic sufferers and if it suits you and you can afford it, try it.

In our wonderful country we suffer from high

humidity, which does not cause rheumatism, but certainly aggravates it. To keep warm and dry we must understand how to combat this dampness. Take a woollen sock which has been dried and well-aired, put it on one hand, hold it in front of the fire for two minutes, and you can feel the dampness going into your hand. This also happens with both your underwear and your bed.

Perhaps our sufferer thinks this is a minor detail, but I assure you that it is another important item in THE WAY OF LIVING. To put on any clothing, or lie on anything which is the slightest bit damp is just asking for trouble. When you do this the body has to dry the article, and doing this drying takes heat and energy from your system. Many people have their bedroom windows open during the day, and close them at night, by which time the bedclothes have absorbed quite a lot of dampness from the atmosphere, and one hot water bottle will not dry a full bed. Whilst it is good health sense to open the windows for one hour at times there is usually quite enough air in any bedroom through all the cracks, gaps and window frames for good breathing. It is not necessary to sleep with windows open in winter, and in chest troubles it is one of the worst things to do. Cold damp air is not helpful in either bronchitis or rheumatism.

Further to the decreasing of vitality by sleeping in dampish beds, many years ago, in the poorer districts, people used to sleep together. Sometimes quite old people slept with a grandchild. It was also said that Granny was looking fine, but poor little Nellie was sickening. This strange occurrence was because Granny was old, cold, and lacking in vitality, and her body attracted warmth and energy from the poor child during the night when everyone is at their lowest ebb.

Elsie was an early middle-aged friend of ours, and after hospital X-rays, a check on her stomach, gall bladder, and almost everything, nothing wrong could be found, but despite this, she was a very sick lady and rapidly deteriorating when she consulted me. Luckily I had local knowledge and it didn't take two minutes to put her back on the road to good health. Her father had died six months earlier, and I discovered that Elsie had been comforting her mother by sleeping with her. Elsie's mother was eighty years old. When Elsie went back to sleeping in a single bed, the immediate improvement in her health was wonderful, and she had no more trouble afterwards.

To sum up this little chapter, we must keep warm and really dry. If you can't sleep with someone younger than yourself, I endorse a good electric blanket, switched on at least two hours before retiring, to dry out your bed thoroughly.

14

BATHS

The skin is an important organ of elimination and this is essential for good health. A very famous doctor once remarked: "All disease is the result of insufficient elimination. Eliminate the poisons and you will be well." We can help the skin by baths of various kinds, and starting with the hot bath I must issue a warning. Too many hot baths are not good for you. They wash away the natural protection of the skin and tend to be rather weakening. The oil in our skin is not only a germ-stopper, but it is also a skin-lubricant, protects the nerve-endings, and plays a vital part in keeping us warm.

If you have two or more hot baths each week, you should replace the lost oil by having an oil bath. This is best taken at night. Go to bed afterwards. It is always better to have your bath at night when you can relax more. Fill the bath with hot water, add plenty of soap flakes to make a good lather, and then pour in four or five tablespoonsful of olive oil. Stir well. When you have soaked in this solution for ten minutes, there will be a lovely feeling of relaxation. All your muscles will feel softer, your joints will feel looser, and most important, every pore is lubricated. This should be done once a month for normal skins, and once a week for dry skins.

Air baths are good for stimulating the skin and restoring tone, thereby helping the skin to react quickly to sudden changes of temperature. With practically nothing on you can potter around the house and do a few chores. At first do this for just a few minutes and as the skin becomes tougher, gradually increase the time.

Bicarbonate of soda baths are for general muscular rheumatism. Put two pounds of bicarbonate of soda in a hot bath. Soak in this for ten minutes, then go to bed with a hot drink and perspire freely. No soap must be used in this bath.

A footbath is the best thing not only for rheumatism, but also for headaches and insomnia if the bath is taken last thing at night. With a large bowl or footbath full of very hot water, mix in two tablespoonsful of powdered mustard and soak the feet for at least ten minutes. All the skin of the body excretes waste matter which is often acid, but none more than the feet. This, I think is because there are more pores per square inch in the feet than elsewhere. People whose feet sweat a lot don't perspire much in other parts of the body, therefore the feet try to make up the balance. After a good soak, when the bottoms of the feet are well softened, try scraping them with your long nails, or a suitable instrument. It is surprising what you can scrape off, and how wonderful your feet feel afterwards.

For all rheumatic sufferers there is a wonderful health aid which can easily be done each week and is beneficial. This is not quite a bath but the friction rub is a great help in improving the circulation. Purchase a nylon scrubbing brush and after cleaning it thoroughly

F

and drying it, start at the feet. Brush upwards towards the heart, with fairly long strokes covering all the skin. Afterwards start at the fingers and brush up the arm to the neck, down the neck as far as possible, and up the stomach, covering the sides and as much of the back as you can, always brushing towards the heart. This is a tonic for your circulation, and the glow and warmth felt afterwards is well worth the effort. There is a tendency to dismiss the skin as a minor organ, but in reality it is the largest organ in the body and it has many functions.

About forty-five years ago two handsome athletes performed on the stage and in the circus ring an exceptional balancing and posing act under the name of The Golden Wonders. These two well-built men were painted in gold from head to foot, and with good stage lighting they looked marvellous. Shortly after the first show, they began to feel unwell, and had to call in a doctor, who soon discovered the cause, and ordered them to remove the gold paint before serious damage was done. Afterwards they had to do this as soon as their performance was over, because their skin could not breathe under the paint. The skin is certainly a most important organ.

15

JOINT POLISHING

In the last chapter we studied skin polishing. Now for a little joint polishing. Most people have seen the beautifully polished end of a ham bone. The end which is a joint is rounded — smooth and shiny with not a blemish. We could say it was polished to perfection. This is how our joints should be, but due to modern civilization we don't live as well as the still natural animals, and often the joint ends of our bones lose their polish, and become rough, dry, and pitted. This is the first sign of early arthritis and is due to lack of movement, lack of lubrication and an acid condition of the bloodstream. The hip joint is often the first to go wrong in the overweight abdominal type, particularly those with tight ligaments.

Seldom do the loose jointed people suffer. The so-called double jointed people (there is no such joint) with longish ligaments, usually suffer more muscle pain than joint pain. With the tight pitted joint, our efforts are directed to obtaining fresh surfaces on the ends of the bones. If you understand polishing or grinding the valves of a car you are half-way to understanding joint polishing.

First we attack the large hip joint with movement. If there is any restriction in the movement of the leg from the hip joint, it is time to get swinging. The movement is a simple leg-swinging exercise trying to keep the movement confined to the leg, and allowing no movement in the back. For the left hip movement, stand with the weight on the right leg, but lean over to the right, resting the right side on a wall or some heavy furniture. Swing the left leg like a pendulum from the hip, with the leg straight — not too far or the back moves. This must be continued for at least one hundred swings, and as it improves, increase to at least three hundred, then try swinging the leg across the front of the body.

Many of my patients have used this exercise and kept their hips free from the crippling stage. In fact Miss Riley was offered an operation to put 'pins' in her hips before the war, but today, in her eighties, she still does her exercise and walks without a stick. After many years of advocating this exercise to hundreds of patients it has taken me years to find a better and easier way to do it. I feel like kicking myself for being so dim.

The new way is to sit sideways, half on a table or bench, with your bad leg hanging loosely down and then swing fore and aft (Fig. 22). This is more comfortable and by restraining movement at the spine and pelvis results are better. To get real results one should do both and many thousands of movements must be done before the joint is restored to some of its former smoothness and the glands begin to secrete their wonderful lubrication.

We can adapt this continuous movement to other joints which are sore or stiff. With the stiff shoulder the same idea of swinging it hundreds of times loosely and not pushing it too far, until one can get the arm

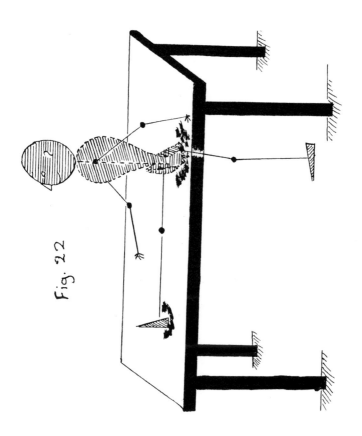

Fig. 22

straight above the head, can be practised. Then, for further improvement, swing the arm backwards in a full circle close to the body. In a very tight shoulder joint, sometimes called a frozen shoulder, one can pull the joint out a little, which not only helps to free it, but allows a little lubrication to flow between the joint surfaces as they open up.

Sit down in a chair and clasp both hands around your knee, which should be lifted a little above the level of the hip with the foot off the floor (Fig. 23). Without pulling with the arms, press strongly downwards with the knee keeping the body perfectly still. The arms must be straight, and the strain is transmitted to the shoulder joint. You will often hear a slight plop, indicating that the joint surfaces have parted.

One joint which can upset the whole of the shoulder girdle is the clavicle sternum, where the collar bone meets the breast bone. When you shrug your shoulders, the collar bone pivots on the breast bone just below the centre of the neck. This is a joint frequently affected by rheumatism, and often missed in diagnosis and examination. Exercise here consists of shrugging the shoulders, lifting them as high as possible, then letting them down relaxed. After this try rolling both shoulders in a backward direction.

Again I must stress that it is only by constant repetition that any real benefit can be obtained. You may as well not bother if you are only prepared to do a couple of dozen. In all my exercises for joint stiffness results come only with multiple movement.

The patient who has difficulty in standing can do this arm swinging while sitting in a chair. The extremities, fingers, toes, wrists, and ankles are

PRESS DOWN
WITH KNEE

Fig. 23

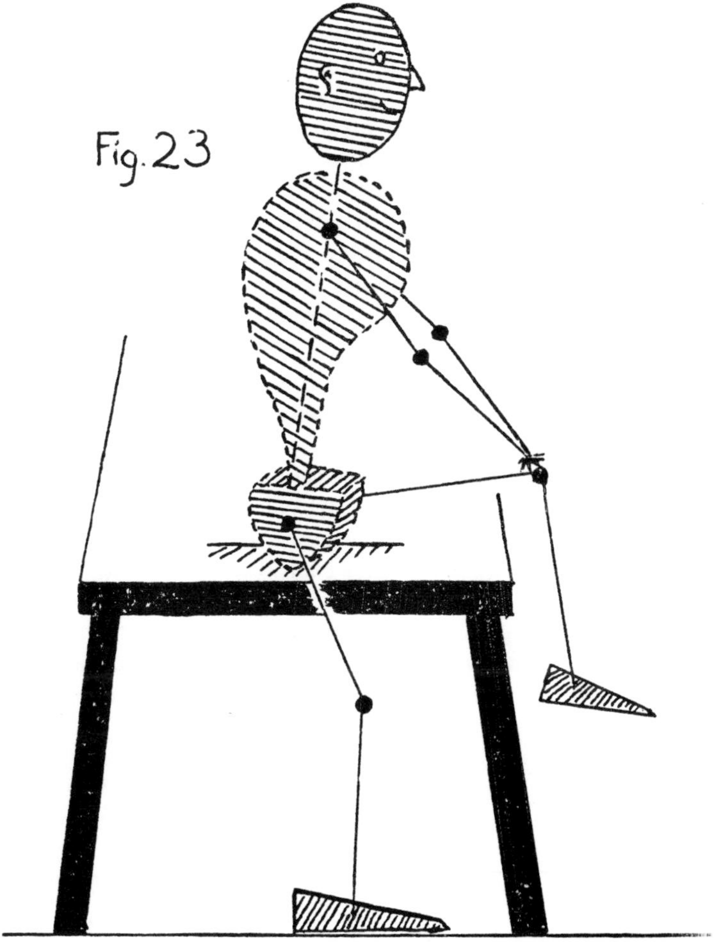

comparatively simple, twisting, turning, rolling, and shaking, opening and closing the fingers, curling the toes, walking on tiptoe and then on the heels. In shaking the arms are held loosely down with the fingers slack. Shake the whole arm from the shoulder for quite a time and feel the blood pulsate into the fingertips.

It is more difficult to shake the leg, but by leaning on the wall or a heavy piece of furniture with your right side you can shake your left leg, then turn and shake the right one.

In improving movement upwards to the neck, here we move the head, and there should be full and easy movement in every direction, but mostly there is restriction in every direction, and so many rheumatic complaints begin in or around the neck that we must mobilize the head. Can you imagine a long distance driver with a free neck? The poor man has no chance to move his head whilst driving, and we find many patients with terribly stiff necks in these circumstances. The remedy is again MOVEMENT of every vertebrae, rolling, turning, and swinging the head in every direction hundreds of times each day. It is possible to do even a quick move or two if you arrive at the traffic lights as they go red. It is possible that the man in the car next to you is doing the same. Many of my patients who drive do this, and I can only hope that it never causes an accident.

The best neck exercise is rotating the head from side to side as though you are trying to look to the right and then to the left, keeping the head at eye level and starting gently, then going further round, moving faster and faster. Your head won't come off but the exercises may make you dizzy, so always sit down for neck exercises.

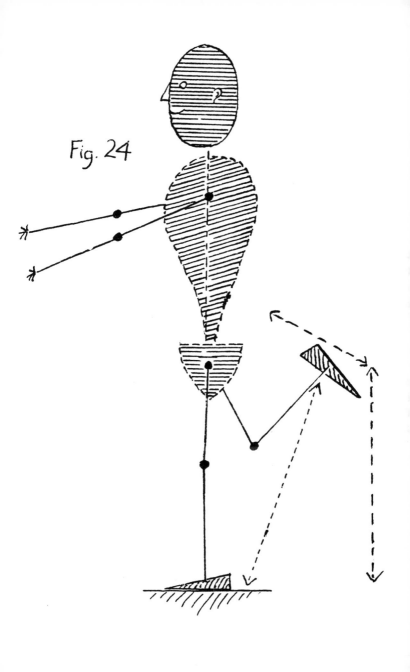

Fig. 24

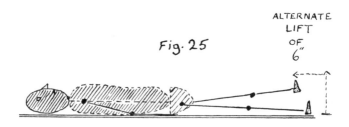

Fig. 25

ALTERNATE LIFT OF 6″

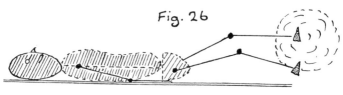

Fig. 26

SMALL CIRCULAR MOVEMENTS

The best exercise of all is walking, and if you can, please try to walk at least two miles each day. People who stand in one position for long hours miss the benefit of walking, and often suffer from poor circulation in the legs, which can lead to varicosity and even worse conditions. Dentists, hairdressers, and other people who must stand practically still for long periods, suffer because it is easy for the blood to flow downwards to the feet, but hard for it to return to the heart. Therefore it is imperative to do something which helps to force the blood upwards, preventing stagnation in the legs. To help we can use the natural venous pump which everyone has in their legs. By lifting the foot backwards as though trying to kick their buttocks with their heels (Fig. 24). This exercise, if done many times, creates a greatly improved upward flow and can be done whilst either at work or at home.

An important asset for circulation, posture and back trouble is good stomach muscles, and we can show just two really good exercises for you. Lie down, face upwards, and try to press the small of the back to the floor. Then lift the legs alternately six inches off the floor, but once started, the feet and legs must not touch the floor until the exercise is over. With the legs perfectly straight, this creates a long lever, which is good for the tummy, but lifting the legs too high spoils the tension (Fig. 25). Whilst in the same position, do a small cycling movement, with very small circles and the legs almost straight, again not touching the floor (Fig. 26).

16

RELAXATION

There are only two basic exercises — concentration and relaxation. If you have mastered concentration, you can soon master relaxation. Muscles which you have exercised with full concentration (thinking of nothing but the part being used) develop tone and are far better than the lesser used muscles. However, let us begin the first lesson. Sit down and bend your left arm to a right-angle in front of you. Put the forefinger of your right hand under your left wrist. Relax the left arm as much as possible, supporting its weight with the right forefinger, and then suddenly remove this digit. What usually happens now is that the left arm is still flexed, or it has dropped just a little and of course it is holding itself in mid-air when, if it had been fully relaxed, it would have followed gravity and fallen limply to your side.

This is the first principle of relaxation and you can practise with any part of the body once you have mastered this with the arms. Keep trying with both arms and ask a friend to give the support, and then remove it to catch you out. Do not force the arm downwards. It must be the weight of the arm assisted by gravity which allows the arm to fall like a stone.

With a little imagination one can apply this to other

parts. Lift up the shoulders for a second, hold them, then relax, and let them fall fully down. Don't push them down. At first you require help to do the legs, and after lying down face uppermost, lift one leg six inches from the floor. Get your partner to put three fingers under your ankle holding all your leg weight. As he suddenly slips his fingers out, your leg should flop to the floor. Don't force it down. Let it fall.

A good semi relaxation for the tired back muscles is to sit on the table with your legs dangling loosely over the edge. Try to sit into the table rather than on it and then swing the legs alternately about twelve inches in front, allowing them to go under the table at the end of each swing. Sitting pretty straight, rest your hands on your thighs, 'sink into' the table, and swing the legs, using an easy pendulum movement with the minimum effort. It takes about four minutes before you feel the relaxation of your back muscles, and I venture to suggest that five minutes' exercise this way will ease many an aching back.

Whilst lying in bed lift each part of the body in turn, and then let it flop down. Lastly lift your head off your pillow, let that flop, and then sink into the bed and forget your pain. Think only of pleasant things, and even if you don't sleep at once it does not matter because you are resting. In any type of rheumatism you should not stay in bed too long. It would be a good idea if we could adopt the old naval idea of four hours on and then four off. The worst stiffness always occurs after six hours.

17

COURAGE

During the war I met quite a number of men with courage, some who received decorations, and many who deserved them, but not one of these heroes had the courage of many of my patients. There are many thousands of severely handicapped people who battle on against frightful odds, and most of these can teach us how to smile and still fight on when life is hard. We should certainly do far more for these deserving triers, and a little less for the able-bodied non-triers. I have been fortunate to meet some of these triers, who deserve a double V.C. at least! Make no mistake, these people don't want sympathy, but a little help and understanding, and we must always remember that they are human beings, above everything else. May I ask your indulgence whilst I give two examples of struggles for existence.

Mr John Salter came to me for treatment in his early forties after suffering for over twenty years from a terrible wasting disease called PROGRESSIVE MUSCULAR ATROPHY. At twenty-one years of age, John weighed ten stones, but at forty he weighed just five stones, and with amazing courage, still worked as a stonemason. He had great difficulty in walking, and at work he had a trestle between his legs to help hold him up erect whilst he cut names on gravestones. He used the swing of his body with his chisel and mallet held close to his chest with both elbows tight into his sides.

If I had not seen him at work I would surely have said that the job was totally impossible for him to do. Can you visualize a man of five feet eight inches at a body weight of five stones, with dreadfully thin arms, being able to cut names in marble all day to support a grand wife and two lovely girls? I marvelled when I saw him at work but even to negotiate a step was a hard task for John. Like most handicapped people, he did not ask for help, but preferred to fight, helped by a wonderful devoted wife and later as his two girls grew up, they could pick him up when he fell which was pretty often. It was not possible for him to get out of a chair without help, but he battled on and continued working cheerfully.

John managed, for a while, to run a small car with spring assisted pedals, and one summer booked a caravan holiday on Anglesey for his family. This was a time of great excitement for his two young girls, and the journey of 130 miles was completed without incident. However, during the first week poor John developed pleurisy, and as anyone knows this is agony, but double agony for people who have little flesh and no padding on their nerve ends. As usual there were no complaints from John and he stuck it out to the bitter end, then he drove his family home and collapsed only when he was in his driveway. What a man!

He had many falls, but one bitter winter's day he fell in Greenacres cemetery, and could not get up without help, so he lay all day in the increasing snow. When he was found by the cemetery keeper at dark almost frozen, he was helped home after refusing to go to hospital.

Eventually he left his stonemason's business, and bought a run-down café on the main Southport road. With his usual grit and determination, and helped by his wife and the now big, strong girls, he made a success of this venture until he passed away at the age of forty-three. He was truly a man in a million.

A few years later his younger daughter came to see me, and I was appalled to discover that she had developed all her father's symptoms. I referred her to the doctor, who said that it was impossible, that the disease was only hereditary in the first-born male, whilst Mary was the second-born female. My reply was that I had also read the textbooks, but after treating Mary's father for years I knew the symptoms.

Mary went into hospital and after tests which confirmed the rough diagnosis an incident occurred in the hospital which was totally wrong. The specialist was discussing the case with quite a group of students around the bed, and said in an easily audible voice: "It's a good thing she doesn't know the end result."

Mary looked up and replied quietly, "I know full well that my father died at forty-three with the disease." When will the great man in hospital start treating us as human beings instead of as numbers? After a short stay in hospital Mary was back at work with her weight falling by about two pounds each week, but she was always cheerful. Later she obtained an Invacar to enable her to get to work.

Eventually she married a fine man, Ian Avison, a lay preacher on the Methodist Circuit. He worked in Huddersfield while Mary worked in Blackley. Ian had to travel about fifteen miles and Mary three, and therefore he was always off to work first, but one morning after he had gone, his wife fell heavily and struck her head on the raised hearth kerb. This did not stop her from going to work, and despite a terrific headache and some vomiting, she managed the day's work, and was making her husband's tea when he arrived home. One look at her was enough for Ian, and a few minutes later at the local hospital, Mary was X-rayed and found to have a fractured skull. No one at the hospital could believe that she had worked all day in this condition.

Some time later when seven months pregnant, she fell and broke her thigh. She did not complain and she had a lovely baby girl, to be followed by another just as lovely two years later. Unable to work any longer, and despite many falls, she not only looked after her family well, but was always helping others. Very seldom did she miss church, and she was carried in by her husband who was very slim, but possessed by strength of body and character because his heart was pure. Even in a very weak state, Mary helped the little children at the local primary school to read, and twelve months before her death she passed an A-level in English. Many people mourned when this lovely courageous girl passed on in her early thirties, and we who intimately knew her will never forget her amazing grit and cheerfulness.

Another patient in my 'hall of fame' is David Foden who contracted polio at the age of seven, and, despite paralysis from the lumbar region downwards, has battled along on crutches and with full calipers to become self-supporting as an accountant and a great sportsman. Whatever it is, David will try it, be it swimming, water polo, table tennis, shot putting, bowls, wheelchair racing, fishing — and smiling. In just over twenty years he has built himself a wonderful body and a superb character. As one of the regular disabled athletes at Stoke Mandevile Hospital's Paraplegic Games, David has won three gold medals, two silver ones and also the award of The Sportsman of the Year, 1973. It is a privilege to treat these wonderful people and feel that you have helped a little. David was allowed out of hospital (Isolation Hospital) by the local orthopaedic surgeon, provided I gave him intensive treatment which I have done for over twenty years, and though he has not always enjoyed it, I have enjoyed treating him. He is the Founder of the Oldham Owls Sports Club for the Disabled, whose members are a very lively crowd of fine people, who don't win a great number of events but are always ready to participate.

18

RHEUMATIC'S PRAYER

"Dear Lord, if I must have rheumatism, help me by Thy divine grace to bear it in such a manner that I do not make every person in the house and elsewhere feel the pain. Give me the courage and grace to refuse to describe over and over again the misery and suffering which belong to me alone. Strengthen in me the desire to get well, that I may not be tempted to live in the pity and sympathy which is often extended to an invalid. May I always remember that pains in the nerves are multiplied by pains in the description of them."

Once again I return to movement. Physical movement is the law of life and the secret of long life. It is essential to impart movement and strength to the organs of the body so that they may perform their functions. Exercise increases the oxygen in the body, produces vigorous circulation, helps elimination, and regenerates the nervous system and vital organs. Constipation, indigestion, nervous complaints, asthma, heart troubles and most other disorders can be improved by taking specific exercise. Physical weakness shows in the drooping posture, round shoulders, flat chest, and lack of tone in all the body muscles. The relaxed stomach muscles bring on constipation and shortness of breath, particularly on exertion. General muscular weakness produces poor circulation, faulty elimination, and general debility of the body. The ultimate end of this weakness is sickness and unhappiness.

It is not possible to be in the best of health unless one takes a certain amount of outdoor exercise. In most forms of chronic disease it greatly contributes to early recovery. Exercise is necessary in becoming well and also in keeping well. Walking is still the finest exercise of all, and as a simple exercise it can be graduated to suit a delicate invalid or a fit athlete improving his heart, lungs and muscular tone. If one can add to this a simple bending and twisting of the trunk, and some deep breathing, you will be rewarded with one of the great joys of living — GOOD HEALTH. Always remember to start gently and gradually progress as the body becomes stronger. Make haste slowly. Just one word of warning. Never exercise until at least two hours after a meal.

19

EXERCISES FOR THE DISABLED
IN WHEELCHAIRS

I am well aware that many disabled people cannot get up and walk, but with a little thought they can often do concentration and isometric exercises, even in a wheelchair. If the arms are unaffected start with neck rolling, shoulder shrugging, and deep breathing, concentrating on forcing out the breath through the mouth, and not allowing any air into the lungs except via the nose. A more vigorous exercise for the neck muscles is to use the hands and press against the head to provide resistance, with your left hand on the left side of your head near the temple, and your head held over to the right as far as possible facing front. Force your head to the left, resisting with the left hand, but just allowing the head to win. Repeat on the opposite side, then try with your head back, and your hand on your forehead, and force your head forwards and down against the push of your hand. Then with both hands clasped at the back of your head, force your head upwards and backwards.

Photo 1 (demonstrated by David Foden)

For arm and chest; clasp your hands in front of your chest with your arms bent, and whilst resisting with the right hand, push with the left, just allowing the left arm to win the push of war. Change to push with your right hand and continue this for a few movements. As with most exercises, it is necessary to do the opposite, and as we have begun by pushing, it is now time to pull, which uses the muscles in a different way. Begin with the same position as before, your hands clasped over to the left, and now pull with your right hand and resist with your left, allowing the pulling right arm to win the tug of war — slowly does it.

Photo 2

Once again use the same position with your fingers interlocked. Grip tightly and pull with both arms, as though trying to open your fingers.

Photo 3

Do the same exercise with your hands over your head. Place your hands over your knees and with straight arms, push onto your knees. Then grip behind your knees and pull upwards. Next put your hands on the insides of your knees and press outwards, followed by putting your hands on the outsides of your knees and pulling inwards. In these exercises one is using muscle against muscle and it can be fairly strenuous at first. You can easily improve by doing a few more repetitions, and no doubt you can experiment with your own exercises on these lines, even pulling or pushing on your wheelchair.

Photo 4

If you can turn your upper body, it is possible to exercise the arm muscles. Turn a little to the left and grip the chair arm with your left hand, keeping the arm as straight as possible, and then try to lift the chair by using your biceps muscle. Hold it for three seconds, then relax. Even though you don't move the chair arm, this concentrated isometric exercise is excellent for the arm flexors, forearm, and grip. Repeat two or three times and then change to the right hand.

Photo 5

Still in the chair, place both hands on the chair arms, and keeping your arms absolutely straight, press hard downwards to raise your body off the chair. Hold this position for three seconds. This is opposite to the previous exercise and develops the triceps and muscles behind the upper arm, and also the shoulders.

With leg movement, pressure is used against the floor or the footrest of your chair. With your right leg stiff and straight, press your heel into the floor. This develops thigh muscles. Again one must hold this position for a few seconds, as this is the real secret of isometric exercises. Repeat with your left leg and as you hold this position it is possible that you can feel your stomach muscles being used.

I realize that many people cannot do these exercises if their bodies are completely paralysed. Can you place one leg over the other and lift this leg upwards whilst resisting with the other? The same idea can be practised by moving sideways and resisting the movement. Next comes bending the knee with the other foot on top of the one you are trying to bend. You can make it hard or easy.

It is possible for some of the disabled to do isometric exercises for the spine. Press your upper back into the chair. Hold this position for five seconds, then relax. Press the lower back likewise, then, turning sideways, press each side in turn, always holding for a few seconds, and then relaxing. There is also sideways and forward bending, without pressure. Tighten the stomach muscles and then hit them with alternate fists. Then do wrist turning followed if possible by ankle turning. Finish by completely relaxing every part of the body that you can. If you feel that you require further graduated exercise, try one with a stick, which gives excellent results once you have acquired the skill of doing it. Obtain a four foot long broomstick. Your first exercise with this is demonstrated by David.

Photo 6 & 7

Press the stick, with your hands shoulder width apart, above your head slowly, as if it weighed at least thirty kilograms. Relax and then repeat, but this time pull outwards as though trying to stretch the stick by making it longer. Repeat, but this time press inwards as though trying to shorten the stick.

Photo 8

Rest, then do the same again, but pushing the stick out in front, again with pushing, stretching, and contracting movements.

Photo 9 & 10

For the biceps, start with your arms straight down, then bend them slowly until the stick touches your chest and repeat, pushing inwards then pulling outwards. These are excellent exercises and they are very useful not only for building muscle, but wonderful for concentration and co-ordination.

Many disabled people can improve their general health by exercising, and in some cases this can improve their circulation so much that their disablement becomes less. While watching disabled sportsmen and sportswomen, one is conscious of their courage, and impressed by the amazing fitness of these wonderful people. These are true athletes who excel at many sports and by exercises and vigorous training have improved their health and strength far beyond the reach of most able-bodied people. I advise the average disabled people who read this book to study the massage movements and if you can do some of them they will surely help.

In stretching contracted ligaments and muscles the patient will experience some pain, which is natural and only to be expected, but keep at it, gently at first, and as the part becomes more supple and stronger the pain will subside. It is hard to begin, and difficult for the handicapped with all their other problems, but try hard and keep on persevering. Not only will your health and strength improve, but you will surely find that as the circulation speeds along through the body, and the brain, the mind becomes more alert, and this will surely help you to a more cheerful approach to your problems.

20

MASSAGE

For the patient with rheumatism who is prepared to treat himself, the first essential is to learn a little about massage technique. Hand massage in rheumatism is at first gentle and soothing, with long gliding even strokes, almost caressing the part, stroking upwards towards the heart, and gradually putting on a little more pressure as you become more used to both the feeling and the movement. The part being treated must always be relaxed, and if possible, supported.
Photo 11
In the picture of David massaging his left forearm from the wrist to the elbow you will notice that the full weight of the left arm is supported by the table. Also note that the wrist is lightly flexed. This stroking can be done with the palm of the hand, the ball of the thumb, or the fingers and it is called EFFLEURAGE (Fig 27). When performing on the limbs try to imagine that you are pressing the blood vessels and emptying them, up towards the heart, as one would with a soft rubber tube which contains water. This same massage movement can be done with the finger and thumb or your fingers, stroking towards the hand and covering the front, back and sides. In working on small digits it is permissible to use quite a strong pressure, with benefit.

106

EFFLEURAGE

Fig. 27

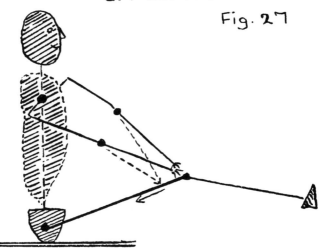

STROKING

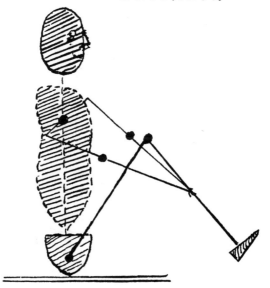

On the legs both hands can be used at the same place, but the part must be supported in a position of relaxation. When doing the lower leg from the ankle to the knee, bend the leg to an angle of 90° if possible, to relax the calf muscle, supporting the weight on a stool (Fig 28). The thigh is covered with the leg straight

Fig. 28

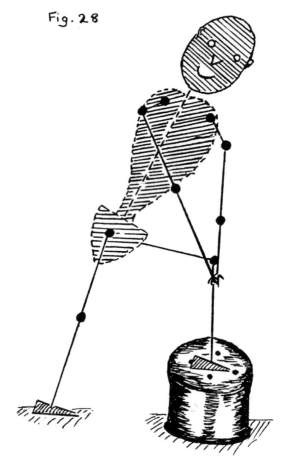

when doing the front, and the leg is bent for doing the back of the thigh. Whenever possible, endeavour to encompass the limb with your hands cupped and thumb on the opposite side of your fingers.

Whilst working on the thigh we can practise the next massage movement, PETRISSAGE (Fig. 29) which is a process of kneading, rolling, lifting, squeezing, and pressing the soft tissues. It can be done with both hands, one hand, both thumbs, or the thumb and fingers. Grasp as much of the relaxed muscle as possible with one hand, squeezing, rolling, and lifting the muscle away from the bone. Release, then grasp again and keep repeating until the muscle appears softer and more relaxed, then move upwards to the next area and repeat, working along the full course of

PETRISSAGE

Fig. 29

KNEADING
ROLLING
SQUEEZING

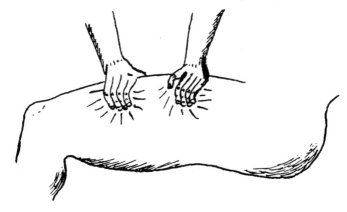

the muscle or limb. With two hands the movement is forwards and backwards in opposite directions. Rollling the muscles is a very good way of muscle manipulation, holding the muscle with both hands and rolling it around the bone, and gradually moving slowly along the limb. Endeavour to knead the muscle as you roll it, and finish with shaking the muscle and all the limb.

These movements should always be followed by easy shaking exercises. If it is the arm which you are shaking, allow it to fall down into gravity and shake the whole limb rapidly from the shoulder until you feel the blood tingling into your fingertips (Fig. 30). This type of massage stimulates the circulation of the blood, nerves, and glands, promotes cell exchange and helps in the disposal of acid and early rheumatic conditions. If only you will have patience and continue your self-massage for a few weeks you will certainly be convinced by the general improvement of feeling, by easier movement with less pain, and as you gain more control of your muscles, so will you be able to relax better. Remember that you cannot stay in one state of health. You go forwards or backwards, and if you do something positive you will certainly go forwards. In the two previous forms of massage use a little olive oil to help smooth the hand movements. You can either put a little on the part to be treated or into the cupped hands.

In the next type of massage we must have the skin completely dry. This is the treatment of choice for all joints, even for arthritic ones. It is also a follow-up of the previous treatments, and my name for this is DRY FRICTIONS (Fig. 31). At first, the patient or student is apt to do large frictions, but one can perform only

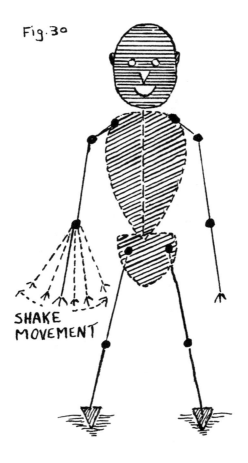

Fig. 30

SHAKE
MOVEMENT

small frictions. Frictions are done with the fingertips or pad of the thumb, but they can be done also with the heel of the hand. The fingers are firmly pressed upon the treatment area and movements made in a circular direction, moving the skin and tissues against the underlying bone. The fingers must not slide over the

FRICTIONS   Fig. 31

LITTLE CIRCULAR MOVEMENTS ON
THE TISSUES AGAINST UNDERLYING BONE
WITHOUT SLIDING OVER THE SKIN

FRICTIONS

FINGERTIP
METHOD

FLAT-HAND
CIRCULAR
MOVEMENTS

skin, but take it along with a small movement. It is
rather like taking up the slack, and besides pressing
down, performing little circles with the operating
finger or thumb.

The chief areas of application are all joints, the
spine, the face and certain nerves. It is really
wonderful for breaking up small adhesions and
loosening tight joints. It is possible to massage all parts
of the spine by frictions with the aid of a belt. I have
taught this method to many patients who live alone,
and I recommend it to you as a wonderful help in all
rheumatic conditions of the back, including lumbago,
sciatica, spondylitis, and muscular pains. The
important part of this useful treatment is that the
frictions must be small movements, with absolutely no
sliding over the skin.

Any type of clean belt will do but it is best to be
about two or more inches wide and fairly long. Strip
off, hope your room is warm, put the belt behind your
back and over your buttocks. Hold one end of the belt
in each hand and pull forwards with both hands to put
pressure at the centre of the belt over your buttocks.
(Illustrated by author photo 12). Now move your
hands alternately forwards and backwards just enough
to move the soft tissues without sliding over them, all
the time maintaining good pressure forwards. Continue up the spine, spending a little time on each part,
keeping the centre of the belt over the spine.

It is often surprising how you will find tender spots
which you didn't appreciate before. Spend more time
on the tender parts, because many pains have their
origins in or around the spinal vertebrae. You may
have pain to one side and it is easy to alter the pressure
from the middle to the side by moving one hand in

H

front of the other. If you require the left side to be treated, all you need to do is to move the left arm forward so that the centre of the belt presses to the left side. For more pressure move the left arm across the front of the body. It is possible to treat every inch of the back and then treat the back and sides of the neck by using your belt, but when approaching the sides of the neck, do not use much pressure. The sides of the neck contain vital glands and blood vessels which should be treated gently. Frictions of the spine are of enormous value in health as well as in rheumatism, and it is worth persevering with your belt as this will help to disperse rheumatic nodules, break down adhesions, remove acid and stimulate the spinal nerves.

Whilst I have always said that there is no substitute for the hands in massage, the belt is a very good second best, and by using it you help your hands and arms somewhat. Given time, and the desire to improve, one can treat every inch of the back with this method which I introduced many years ago, and I myself benefited from it in my early arthritic days.

Frictions on joints that one can reach are just marvellous. Let us take a left wrist which is tight and painful. If there is no severe inflammation or extreme swelling we can begin, using the middle fingers of the right hand, with small circular frictions from the base of the fingers, slowly working up past the wrist, covering every inch of the area, and including the palm of the hand. The left hand must be supported on a table, and as relaxed as possible, with the patient sat comfortably. Having completed massaging the back and front of the hand, half turn the wrist and work on the side of the wrist and thumb. Turn again and complete the little finger side, always resting the hand fully on the table.

Because the muscles which control the wrist and finger movements are in the forearm we now treat this area from the wrist to the elbow using first the stroking technique, then squeezing, rolling and lifting the muscles, and finishing by frictions aimed particularly at the area around the muscles just below the elbow joint. The forearm must be resting on the table and a little extra friction should be given on the elbow joint. You can often find soreness around here, and as with other tender spots you must concentrate on these to get the greatest benefit. For the upper arm the best movement is stroking with your thumb on one side, and your cupped fingers on the other, then changing to one on top and the other below, pressing up towards the shoulder and squeezing a little.

All this work gives a fair amount of exercise to the fingers on the hand used, and it is now necessary to treat the fingers and thumb individually. Stroke from your nail to your palm, covering the sides as well as the front and back using your thumb and first two fingers. Then do frictions on each knuckle with your thumb on top and finger below; the main effort is by thumb-circling and pressing into all the joints. I realize that this takes time and energy, and it is possible to spend ten to fifteen minutes really doing one arm, from finger to shoulder, but you are not required to cover the whole body at one session. In fact, you ought to concentrate mostly on the painful areas, though it is not always at the painful spot that the trouble originates.

Many painful arms and hands can be caused by stiffness in the back of the neck, with the pain radiating down the nerves. The same is applicable to the leg when there is tightness in the lower back and the more we study the body, the greater our realization of the terrific importance of the spine and the necessity of treatment and exercise here.

There are three important muscles at the top of the arm that form the shoulders. These are the anterior deltoid muscles and the lateral and the posterior deltoid. As the name explains, the anterior helps to lift the arm in front of the body, the lateral lifts sideways, and the posterior moves the arm backwards. In fibrositis of the muscle or in arthritis in the shoulder joint, these muscles tend to waste, because it is painful to lift the arm, and some massage devoted to this area, followed by local exercise, will work wonders. Sit on a low stool and rest the whole of your arm on a table. This is the position of relaxation for the deltoids, and now you can give firm stroking to them, followed by frictions using three fingers of the other hand. If you press your arm down on the table you will find that the anterior deltoid becomes soft and relaxed, and while it is in this condition you can pinch and knead this important muscle. This muscle tends to waste rather quickly in conditions where it is difficult to move and lift the arm, e.g. frozen shoulder and most strokes.

The exercise after massage is simple swinging movements many times, stopping short of the painful range. It is neither good nor necessary to swing too far. With the arm held down allow it to swing gently and loosely like a pendulum. When your shoulder has become a little freer try 'walking up the wall'. Stand about six inches from a wall and place the fingers of your bad arm on the wall, level with your waist. Then, using your fingers like very short legs, walk up the wall, pressing a little into it. Go as high as you can and then repeat. If you can ask someone to mark the highest point you reach, you have now a guide for your future progress. Try to climb up higher each day, and when the pain eases, press some of your body weight forward as you get the arm to reach its top limit. This forces the arm further back and is as good as manipulation.

Massage for your neck begins with stroking down the back and sides with four fingers, then frictions with the tips of three fingers, finishing with gentle squeezing of the sterno mastoid muscles which are on each side of the neck. You can bring the left one into prominence by turning your head to the right, then gently squeezing the belly of the muscle from behind the ear to the breast bone, using the thumb and forefinger. Use the same digit to move the Adam's apple from side to side, then stroke from your chin to your breast bone.

All facial massage must be done gently with small circular frictions, concentrating on every sore part. It is possible even to improve the digestion with cheek massage which stimulates the digestive glands in the mouth. Once again, after massage we must exercise. Move the lower jaw from side to side, open the mouth wider than usual, make funny faces, and blow out the cheeks. This all helps to disperse the rheumatism that you can have anywhere, even behind the eyes. Every inch of the face can receive friction massage — this is not beauty treatment, although with a good facial massage followed by the application of hot towels, even if you don't look more beautiful, you will certainly have more colour and feel much better.

You naturally work on all the painful spots, and the surprising discovery of many of these that you did not know existed until you began your frictions. If there is pain or soreness then there is acid (almost certainly rheumatic acid) below the skin. The acid can be dispersed into the circulation with facial frictions. Friction massage the forehead by using three fingers of each hand to wrinkle the skin fairly vigorously. Close your eyes, and using two fingers do gentle frictions over the lids, then use frictions which are a little stronger around the eye socket. Put one finger into the inner corner of the eye and use tiny frictions, including the top of the nose, which often becomes blocked by catarrh or rheumatism. The tiny frictions tend to keep open the small channel which allows surplus tears to drain into the nose.

Another part which tends to stiffen with rheumatism is the angle and joint of the lower jaw, just below the ear. Use three fingers here and cover the front of the ear. Open and close the mouth whilst working on this part. Gentle suction of the ears is performed with the little finger pushed into the ear and quickly vibrated inwards and outwards. Try to keep the finger airtight with the sides of the aperture. If the little finger is tiny, use the next one. This treatment is quite effective by the tiny gentle suctions and stretch on the eardrum.

You can use the palm of the flat hand for the lower jaw. Use your finger and thumb for the upper lip and the nose. Now grasp the end of your nose and shake it really vigorously. After all this work soak a face cloth in hot water, wring it out and apply it to the whole of your face a few times. You cannot appreciate the lovely feeling of full facial massage until you have experienced it. You have now stimulated the circulation locally, stimulated the digestive glands in the mouth, and loosened the jaw, and you should feel a little improvement in seeing and hearing.

Chest massage is mainly to move or manipulate the ribcage and loosen the chest muscles, again the choice is dry frictions, using the full hand, but just the fingertips over the breast bone. Finish by carefully pressing the bottom of the breast bone inwards four or five times. You should be able to move this bone at least half an inch, when it will spring back. Do the same with the ribs, starting at the sides and finishing at the front with frictions performed by the full arm of each hand.

To increase the elasticity of the ribs cross the arms in front of the chest, with your fingers spread under your armpits, then as you press inwards with the hands, press likewise with the forearms as though giving yourself a hug. Move gradually downwards until you have sprung every rib, using less force as you get lower. To open the ribs we sit down, place both hands on top of our head, take a deep breath, hold it, then bend sideways from the waist, first to the left and then to the right. This really opens the ribs on each side and takes the pressure off the intercostal nerves which run between each rib. They can be very painful when they are trapped between ribs. Intercostal neuritis is the name for this complaint, and many times it can be cured by one ten-minute session of rib-opening.

Abdominal massage is of great importance in treating constipation, by stimulating the peristaltic action of the bowels, invigorating the muscular abdominal walls and mechanically pushing along the contents of the intestine. Never massage the tummy just after a meal, never in pregnancy or in any painful inflammatory condition. It is also unwise in high blood pressure, as it can lift the pressure by twenty points. Empty the bladder before you start. The abdomen must be fully relaxed, and it is only possible to do this by lying face upwards on the floor with your knees drawn up, your feet on the floor, and a cushion behind your head. Using the palm of your hand, start at the bottom right-hand side and firmly stroke up the right side across the top of the tummy to the upper left side, then firmly down the left side, moving a little to the midline as you get lower. This is following the large intestine, and to help along the contents continue a few times with increasing pressure. Now using both hands, roll and squeeze the abdomen, kneading with the heels of the hands and dipping the fingertips into the muscle or fat. A useful practice is to do this each time you are on the toilet — AN EXCELLENT HABIT.

21

FEET

The human animal is almost the only animal which cannot stand when born, and in the twelve months or so that it takes Super Man to learn to walk, deformities of the feet have been instituted by ignorance or neglect. The first mistake is overfeeding and the bonny heavyweight child throws terrible strain on its feet while they are developing. Next we have woollen socks which shrink when washed, press the toes inwards and often shorten the tender foot. Later on in life we have that strange thing called fashion which, for reasons I can never understand, must be followed. Some of the shoes worn today will surely make many foot cripples tomorrow, and the effect of these shoes can unbalance the whole body. Without a doubt, when the feet are painful the rest of the body suffers, and today many older people are suffering from bunions, chilblains, metatarsalgia, arthritis and numerous foot troubles due to early neglect.

Once again the main effort is prevention and parents should endeavour to prevent overweight, stop their children from wearing overtight foot apparel, encourage movement of the ankles, feet and toes, dry the feet well and anoint them with olive oil. In later foot troubles I find that many people tend to wash and soak their feet to ease the pain. This is all very good except that the hot water and soap remove the natural oils which are a wonderful protection, and vital to the soft pads under the feet. It is these fibrous and fatty cushions which separate the bones from the sole, and enable the feet to bear enormous pressure. Once again the overweight person puts far greater strain on his feet, which have to support all the weight of his body. This is a terrific task. Is it any wonder that they complain?

Many people have flat feet. In some people it is hereditary and may never cause any trouble. Quite a percentage of native runners are flatfooted but they can run for mile after mile, often without shoes. Over fifty per cent of people in this country suffer from foot troubles, ranging from slight bunions to severe arthritis in every joint of the toes, ankle and foot.

Frequent conditions are athlete's foot or Bengal foot rot, where the foot becomes infected after the skin loses its suppleness and cracks, particularly between the toes. Why athletes, and why is the trouble so prevalent in Bombay and Calcutta? In my opinion it was because of too frequent washing of the feet with soap and hot water. Many athletes have a greater tendency to perspire due to their extra exertions, and they wash away the natural oils with the resulting dry cracking of the skin, and infection often picked up from the gymnasium floor or the swimming pool. The Bengal foot rot condition is identical, and due to the hot weather and also the wearing of shoes and socks, combined with washing the hot feet perhaps three times a day, is it any wonder that the skin dries out? When the skin cracks many people suffer further from the dye of the socks getting into the broken skin. This is mostly applicable to white people, for I never saw a native, who was barefoot, with the rot. He seldom washed his feet with soap and hot water, and he usually walked whilst we sat in cars.

There are, of course, exceptions, and I have treated some of these but the finest example of good feet belonged to one of my famous patients, Lt.-Col. R. Crawshaw, O.B.E., T.D., D.L., M.P., who with great courage and determination improved his health by exercise. Mr Crawshaw is a modest man, and I could relate many of his outstanding feats, but I will just record his letter to me, as it gives a very slight insight into his life.

June 15th 1977. His present age is 59. At the age of eight, he had rheumatic fever and a recurrence at 14 years old. He had pneumonia three times before the age of 5. He later indulged in exercise because, he said, "The doctor said it would kill me — but it didn't." He served in the Parachute Regiment during the war and he is still on reserve as a Colonel. He took up long distance walking by chance and was asked to do a 52 mile marathon, decided to join in at the last minute and came third. Later he broke the world record for non-stop walking (he had three limited stops, each of five minutes). This increased his record from 231 to 255 miles (1972). He still holds the ABSOLUTE non-stop world record of 231 miles without a single stop. He has raised more than £16,000 for charity in the past five years, and he can cure most troubles by exercise, firmly believing that 90% of the illness is mental, rather than physical, and that a determined effort can cure it. He thinks that most of the medical profession does not fully understand the human body. Unless a bone is broken they are often unable to diagnose the complaint. They have little knowledge of the side effects that a displacement can have, and the National Health Service could save millions of pounds each year if they had people who could understand these matters. Many sufferers are at present being treated for the wrong complaints.

Once again we have a fine example of exercise not wearing out the body. I can assure you that Mr Crawshaw has wonderful feet and legs which show no signs of wear and tear. How much longer must we listen to the so called specialist telling us: "It's wear and tear and you must rest"? Rest produces rust, and even if the body could wear out that is better than its rusting away. When the body requires rest, nature tells us in no uncertain terms, and if we push ourselves beyond a certain mark, we faint, or even black out but this is only in extreme cases.

Study your body and so often you will find that tiredness comes on when you have to do a disagreeable task, and very seldom do you feel tired when you are getting ready for, and looking forward to a good holiday. I implore you to keep moving and do it cheerfully.

Apart from the nose the big toe is the coldest part of the body, and the lack of circulation here can aggravate any weakness in this part. It is necessary to move to help this difficult circulation. The blood flows into the legs. This flow is helped by gravity and pushed down by the pumping of the heart, so one can see how easy it is for the arterial blood to reach the feet. However it is a far more difficult task for the blood to return upwards to the heart via the veins. This really is an uphill journey, helped a little by various valves in the veins, but relying mostly on the suction of the diaphragm and the contraction of the leg muscles. Again we must appreciate that without movement the circulation in the legs stagnates more than the circulation in any other part of the body. Most of the swollen legs and feet we see are due to the blood and fluid which does not return fully to the heart. If this is not improved by movement and medicine, we can be burdened by varicose veins, phlebitis, ulcers and in extreme cases, occlusion which could necessitate amputation.

Sometimes we find a patient with the circulation in the left leg restricted while the right leg circulation is quite good. This is often caused by lower bowel distention, constipation, flatulence or swelling in the left groin. The explanation is that the femoral vein, which takes the blood up into the left vena cava passes close to the left lower bowel and any increase in this part of the intestine presses on the vein, restricting the venous flow. On the right side we have a cut away on the intestine near the appendix and there is usually no pressure on the returning blood here. If you have any inflammation or soreness in either vein ulcers or any suggestion of phlebitis, definitely do *not* massage, but consult your doctor. He can prevent the dangerous blood clots and if necessary, can give you tablets to thin the blood, and check for sugar which can be a great complication in leg troubles.

What can you do? Plenty — if you are prepared to try. First, approach the left groin to reduce the swollen intestine which is restricting the venous flow. With your left leg raised as high as possible apply heat just above the thigh. (A hot water bottle will suffice). Gently stroke the vein on the inside of the thigh from the knee upwards to the groin four or five times, leaving the leg raised and using the palm of the left hand. This is the first effort to help the blood to flow to the heart. Afterwards we must reduce the swollen intestine, and the method is cold compress (to contract). Take a large face cloth dipped in ice-cold water and squeezed out, and then fold it to about the size of your hand. Place it over the left lower bowel four inches above the left groin. Cover with a large towel and leave for about four minutes. Repeat three or four times, and then make an effort to contract all the stomach muscles by tensing as one would when bearing down. Further strengthening of this part is by gently hitting it with the inside of the clenched fist. If you wish to you can do this all over the stomach muscles. About a dozen slaps will help to tighten and contract the outer muscles which always stimulates and tightens the muscles of the intestine.

Most bowel distention is caused by weak stomach muscles and flatulence. Any trunk exercises will strengthen the muscles, but the cure for flatulance is by diet and charcoal biscuits. Charcoal biscuits will absorb 200 times their bulk of gas which helps a lot, but let us try not making too much gas by eliminating these gas-forming foods: ALL FRIED FOODS, PEAS, BEANS, CABBAGE, CAULIFLOWER, ONIONS, CUCUMBER, NUTS and SPICES, and by chewing food much more slowly, by not eating or drinking very hot meals, by trying not to drink with meals and by taking half a glass of ice-cold milk at the end of each meal. In a further effort to assist the return blood flow from both legs, raise the bottom of your bed three inches with a couple of blocks of wood. This raised foot of the bed allows the stagnant blood to flow slowly upwards whilst one sleeps, and not only helps to reduce swelling in the legs and feet but also stops a great deal of cramp. If only we could stand on our heads for a few sessions each day we would certainly have much less leg and foot trouble, and far, far better general circulation.

My earlier leg-bending exercise is necessary for circulation here and so is repeated foot movement, but the greatest stimulant for leg circulation is from the DIAPHRAGM. I will try to teach you control and breathing from the diaphragm. The lifting of the diaphragm stretches the large veins which go through to the heart, bringing back the blood which has done wonderful work on our legs. It acts as a marvellous suction pump, and learning to control this action can produce a superb feeling of fitness. Diaphragm breathing is a little difficult to learn, but the effort is more than worthwhile.

In normal breathing we inhale by lifting the chest, opening the ribs, and filling the upper part of the cavity. Very few people use the bottom of the lungs fully. Therefore we have a lung condition where the residual air in the lowest part is almost stagnant, and this mixed with phlegm can be a source of infection and disease. How soon before this develops into shallow breathing and later bronchitis, with all the complications. Because there is lack of mobility in the chest we often find rheumatism encroaching in the part. Many of you have been taught how to breathe, and deep breathing is good, but with the addition of Diaphragmatic breathing, not only will your health improve but your leg circulation will certainly speed up far more than you can believe. Less cold feet, less cramp, less-tired legs, and less danger of ulcers, varicose veins, phebitis or occlusions will result.

Without doubt the improved circulation will make a decided improvement in your rheumatic legs and feet. Your lesson is now explained and I do hope that you can follow the instructions and continue the exercise daily.

Stand against a wall with your back resting on it. Place your left hand in the centre of your abdomen just below the bottom of your breast bone. Practice a few times without breathing, pushing in with the flat hand, and pushing the upper tummy out against light pressure of your hand. There must be no movement of the chest or ribs. Now for the real exercise. Breathe in and force the air to the bottom of the lungs, pushing the upper tummy out against light hand pressure, filling the diaphragm and forcing it down and forwards. This is the opposite to ordinary breathing, and you must try not to move the ribs at any time in Diaphragmatic breathing. When you can do this fairly easily dispense with the hand pressure (photos 13 and 14).

This type of breathing is an enormous help in endurance and it also relieves tension in the nervous system. The centre of the sympathetic nervous system is the solar plexus and it is situated behind the stomach in front of the spine. By pushing the diaphragm forward this has a definite relaxing effect on the nervous system. It is rather difficult to explain why this is so, but having seen the results of this exercise on many patients of a nervous disposition, I am convinced. All good singers learn this type of breathing. They are usually a healthy group and seldom suffer from nervous complaints.

Once again I ask you, what this has to relate it to the feet? The reply is that you cannot separate one part of the body from another. They are all interdependent and, as I repeat, the lifting of the diaphragm, the deep breathing and the stimulating of the heart help the blood supply to the feet. Without this blood supply, we would be sorely tried. Before we get right down to the feet, there is one important muscle which we must treat first — the TIBIALIS ANTICUS, (why ever do they still use these stupid names?) which lifts the front of the foot at the ankle, and any weakness of this muscle allows the foot to drop. This often happens after a stroke and in people who have been in bed a long time. This muscle, situated on the outside of the shin bone, runs down from just below the knee and finishes under the inside of the foot. It is a very hard muscle (shin meat) and can be a real rheumatic scourge, but it responds to deep massage better than any other muscle in the body. It is the one place that you can really dig in without fear of doing any damage and the muscle will readily respond to a simple lifting exercise.

Sit on a chair without shoes and knees fully flexed, with your feet flat on the floor. Lift your foot as high as possible, keeping your heel on the ground. If you take size eight shoes you should be able to lift the front of your foot six inches off the ground — measure to straight big toe. If you are much lower than this there is restriction at the ankle or weakness at the tibialis anticus muscle. This simple exercise should be done for at least fifty movements, and afterwards treat the muscle hard with deep frictions using two or three fingers and concentrating on any sore spots — you will often find them here. Whilst digging in try to move the muscle sideways and outwards away from the (tibia) shin bone. It is best done sitting on a stool with your

J

foot flat on the ground, and with your knee bent to about 90°.

FOOT AND ANKLE. Many people have tightened achilles tendons and you can easily test yours to find out if they are tight. If you cannot raise the foot as we did in the last exercise it could be the tendon at the back of the heel which is tight. This is discovered by gripping the tendon three inches above the heel with your thumb and forefinger. If the tendon is sore and feels tight you have a strained achilles tendon which could be rheumatic, and the cure is to massage with your finger and thumb, and then gradually stretch the tendon by pulling the front of the foot towards you with the leg straight, as you have possibly seen the footballers do when they have cramp in the calf muscle.

To improve the ankle movement and help disperse rheumatic acid which tends to adhere around these bones, use dry frictions with three fingers probing between the joint spaces. Then stroke from the toes upwards, both above and below the foot. Next try to grip the bones approximate to the toes (the metatarsal bones), using both hands with your fingers below your foot and your thumb on top trying to separate one bone from its neighbour by lifting one up as you push the next down. Grip tightly, pulling and pushing until you feel some freedom between each bone, and often you can get a crack denoting a break of adhesions which have been binding two bones together. With the toes, use small frictions and then grip each in turn, stretch as though trying to make them longer, then twist, turn and bend them in every direction. Pay particular attention to the big toe and try to loosen it as much as possible.

In all these manipulations it is vital that the first movement you do is a stretching one to open the joint, and the grip here is by finger and that precludes any massage, or movement around the big toe. This condition is gout. Gout is a very painful affliction mainly attacking the big toe which becomes terribly inflamed and swollen with crystal deposits in the joint. It is generally caused by the overeating of acid forming foods and generally too rich living, more often in men than in women and one could say affluent men. The main reason why the big toe is attacked is that it is the coldest joint in the body. There are drugs your doctor can give you to help the joint, but unless you cut down on the acid forming foods such as alcohol, heavy meats, pork, pastry, fried foods, offal, white bread, sugar, salt, spices and condiments, you will not respond very much. Some people with gout cannot tolerate apples, but all gout patients can benefit by eating grapes, grapefruit (without sugar) raw carrots, pure unsweetened pineapple juice, celery, and bran.

With all circulatory trouble in the lower regions we must avoid all restrictions, suspenders, garters, body belts, tight socks and tight shoes.

22

SUMMARY

To sum up or analyse the previous pages is now our task. The true art of healing is a system of cure which removes the cause of the disease and assists the vitality to correct injury and restore normality. Nature can be depended on to cure, once all the causes are removed.

Is your cause WORRY?

Is your cause OVEREATING?

Is your cause LACK OF MOVEMENT?

Is your cause *a combination of all three*?

Could it be a *lack of faith*, and a generally pessimistic mental attitude?

The health of the human body depends on the health of the billions of minute cells which compose it. These cells have to be magnified hundreds of times before we can see them. Yet they are independent living beings which feed, grow multiply and die like the big cell man. These wonderful cells which make up the whole body perform their individual functions. Some manufacture chemicals, some control foods, others are excretory, and they all work without our conscious aid. It is a most wonderful system and one can only marvel at the superb interrelation between the billions of cells doing vastly different work. All their activities appear to be controlled by the

132

sympathetic nervous system. They are in direct communication with the brain, and every impulse is conveyed to the brain. If there is confusion or dismay in the mind, this is passed over the nerve trunks and filaments to every cell in the body, resulting in the disorganization of the working cells, and thus the vital processes of the human organism, digestion, assimilation, elimination, respiration and circulation of the blood, which normally are completely involuntary, become disturbed.

Think carefully before you give way to worry, please don't let your mind damage your body. Every wrong thought is going to cause some little upset in your cells but conversely, every good thought and deed produces a new harmony. Cultivate a more cheerful disposition and smile more. It doesn't cost anything. Make every effort to replace negative, dismal thoughts by pleasant ones. Always keep in your mind the definite knowledge that the body is always striving to improve your health. Have faith in NATURE and also in YOURSELF — think positively and look for the good in others and in life. To help forget your worries, try doing something for someone. It will help you to stop worrying for a while and give you a general feeling of having done well. Anxiety, tension and stress are a part of life, but unless you control them they can become killers, causing blood pressure to rise, and certainly making your rheumatism worse. Without any doubt they do cause a chemical imbalance in the body cells. There is no perfection in this life, but there is always room for improvement, mentally, physically, and spiritually. It is not what happens to a person, but how his body reacts to the occasion.

The man in the Far East arrives home to find his

house burned down, his family lost, and all his possessions gone. He does not become hysterical, nor does he secrete pints of acid poison from his suprarenal glands and others. He kneels down facing East and says, "It is the will of Allah." Despite this terrible tragedy he remains calm and does not damage his body, because he has FAITH and he really believes.

If only we could have such faith when visited by tragedy how much better we would be in every way. Can you try to cultivate more faith in your friends, neighbours, relations, in nature and in God? Every emotion, every thought has a direct effect upon the physical body. Discord in the mind is translated into physical disease, whilst hope, faith, cheerfulness, happiness and love create HEALTH.

23

FOOD AND MOVEMENT

The purpose of food is to sustain the body and help replace tissue which is broken down by exercise and other factors. We must eat to live, not live to eat, or just gratify our desire for the nice things. The tendency today is to make food as artificial and pleasing to the eye as possible without any heed to its health value. There is too much refining and demineralizing of foods, i.e., white bread, white sugar, polished rice, barley, lentils, preserved meats and fish, sweetened jams, fancy cakes and chocolates.

Too much boiling and frying of foods, i.e. boiling of vegetables kills the valuable salts and their health-giving properties. Natural foods are the essential ones needed for the perfect functioning of the human body. All natural foods, taken fresh from the earth plant, tree or animal, contain the elements necessary for health. If each day we can eat a fresh salad, composed not just of a little lettuce, but of all the raw food in season, such as grated raw carrot, grated raw cabbage, celery, mint, watercress, onions, cauliflower and spinach we have acquired an abundance of vital life-giving minerals.

The vitamins are supplemented by daily fresh fruits. These foods are the basis of good health, and if only one can eat these foods, and less of the acid-forming foods, you are on the way to feeling the best thing possible — VITAL PULSATING HEALTH. After the age of 25 growing has completely stopped, and as the human animal grows it requires a fair amount of food, but after 25, much less is required. It is at this period that people begin to suffer from overeating, and their health starts to deteriorate. If you really desire good health choose the right foods and EAT LESS as you grow older.

If you want to be fit, always be hungry and never, never fill your stomach. The average stomach holds about 1½ pints of liquid, and when you eat the valve at the base of the stomach closes to hold the food inside the stomach until digestion is well on its way. Just imagine what happens when someone eats a rather big meal and at the same time drinks a pint of fluid, as I have often seen them do. With the food more or less converted into liquid, added to the fluid taken, plus the digestive juices, we have two pints in a container which only holds 1½ pints. What happens? The poor stomach distends, often pressing on the diaphragm, even to the base of the heart, causing heartburn, indigestion, discomfort, flatulence and poor digestion.

The stomach is the powerhouse of the body, and if we continually overload it, we will surely 'blow a fuse', and body fuses are not easily repaired. How can you expect this slurpy overfull stomach to perform the difficult task of digestion? We see people eating and drinking far too much, and practically starving in a land of plenty, because the overloading prevents the food from being perfectly digested, and only well-digested food can be assimilated into the bloodstream. You must know of people who are losing weight despite pushing down an enormous quantity of food. Many of my patients in this category have reduced their intake by over fifty per cent and started to gain weight.

Lack of movement is a tragic condition which allows the body to become stiffer and stiffer, slowing down the circulation, and in time we have both physical and mental stagnation. When an animal is in good physical condition it is forever on the move, exercising in a natural way for the sheer joy of living. Watch the lively kitten and note that the more it runs, jumps and rolls the fitter it becomes. The same applies to the young puppy, and to a lesser extent the healthy child, but just a little too much food makes its liveliness slow down. As the child becomes fat, movement is less and less, starting a train of sluggish living which can be a curse for the rest of its life.

When the stomach is empty one has more energy and the desire to move is greater. Movement begets movement, and once you start the effort becomes easier each time. Can you walk one hundred yards? If so do it once every day for the first week, and twice daily for the second and you will easily walk two hundred yards the third week. Keep it up, increasing the distance and the number of times daily, and in six months you will walk two miles with ease.

Walking is the finest of all exercises and if only you will do progressive walking your HEALTH WILL IMPROVE. Combine a little deep breathing with walking, forcing the air out through the mouth, and making sure that the fresh air comes in only through the nose. Try to hold a good posture, and step out to the best of your ability. Take that frown off your face and smile at the world. You are your own master and you are in charge of your own health. The responsibility is totally yours. It is your duty to both yourself and your family to do your best and to improve your health. Only you, helped by nature, can effect a remarkable change, and slowly but surely turn the vicious circle from poor health to the opposite circle, toward GOOD HEALTH.

If you have done very little exercise for years it is best to take it easy at first and expect some soreness the next day. If there is no soreness the day after exercise, we usually say you haven't done enough. As you progress, this soreness, or muscle fever as we call it, will become less and less, although doing a completely different exercise will often bring it on again. Don't let a little pain put you off. Grit your teeth and have a go. DON'T BE A NONTRIER. HAVE FAITH AND *MOVE*.